AF180937

Nonalcoholic Fatty Liver Disease - An Update

Edited by Emad Hamdy Gad

Published in London, United Kingdom

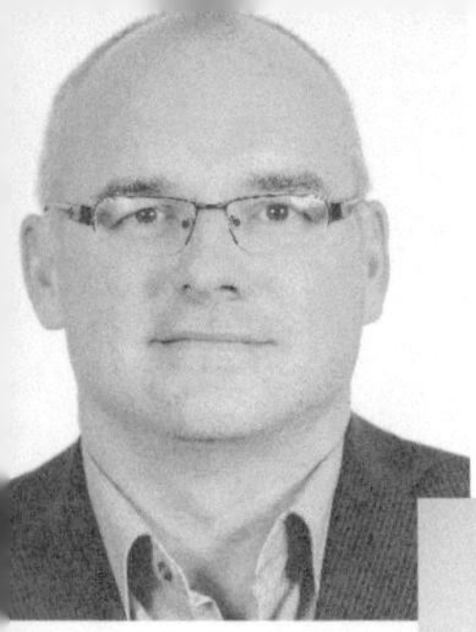
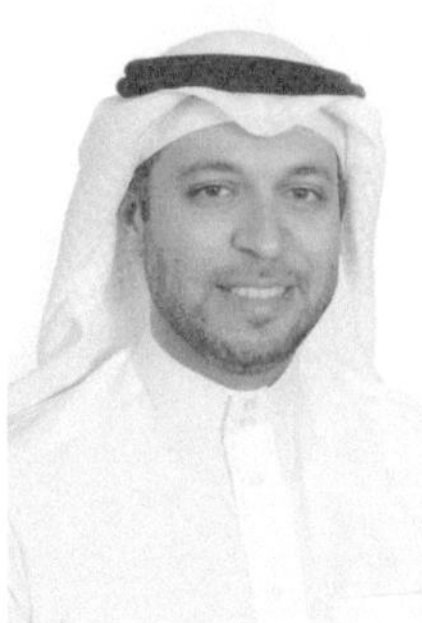
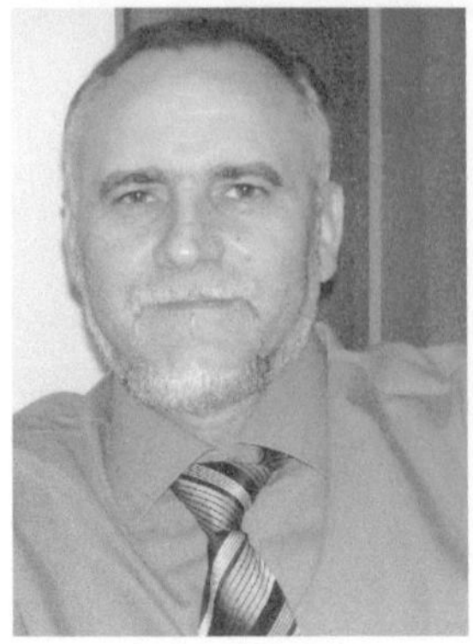
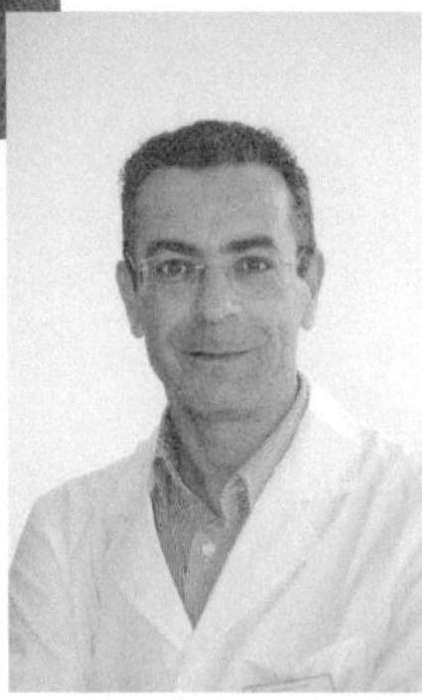
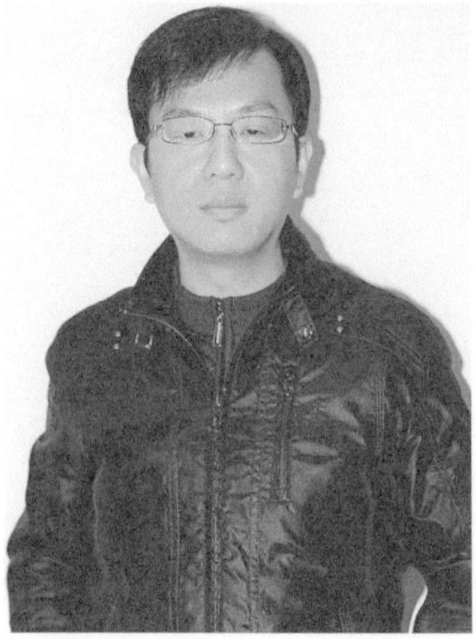
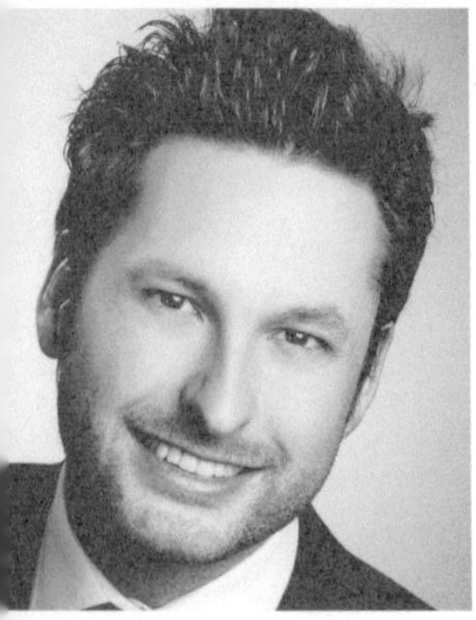
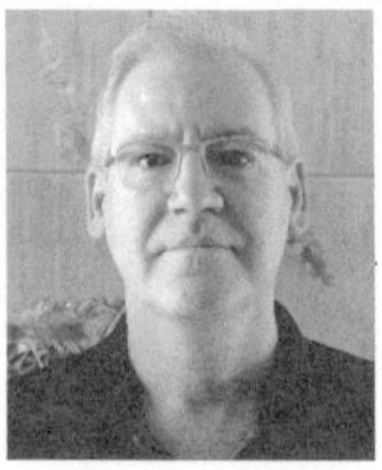
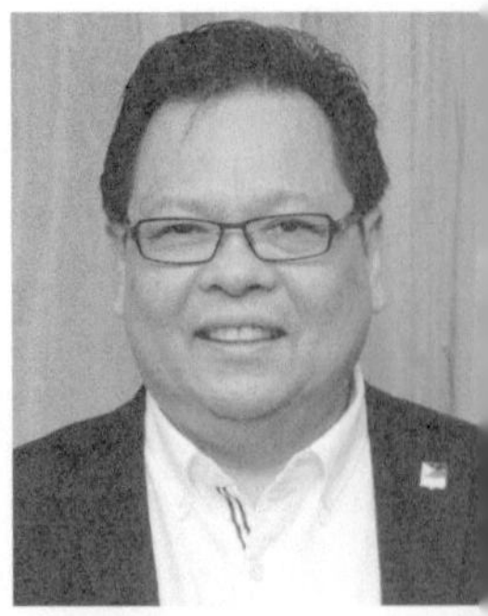
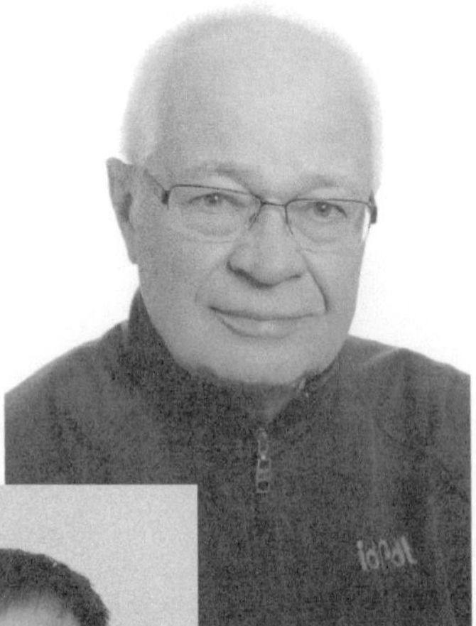
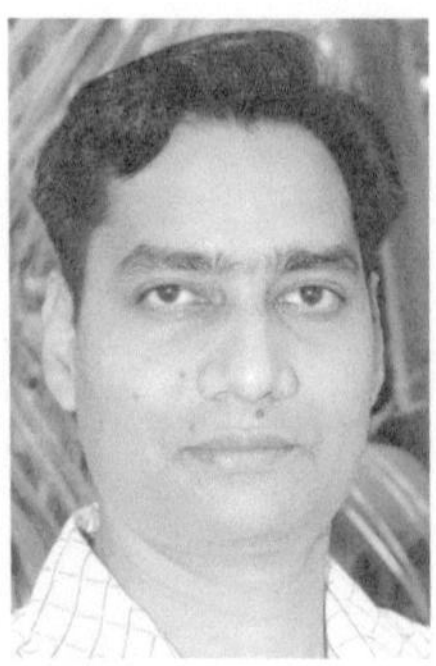
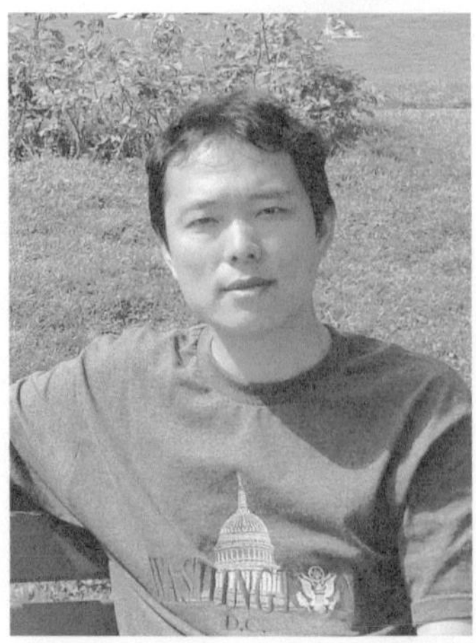
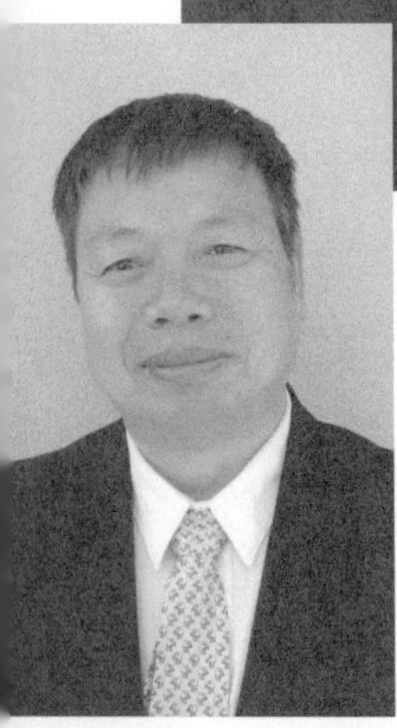
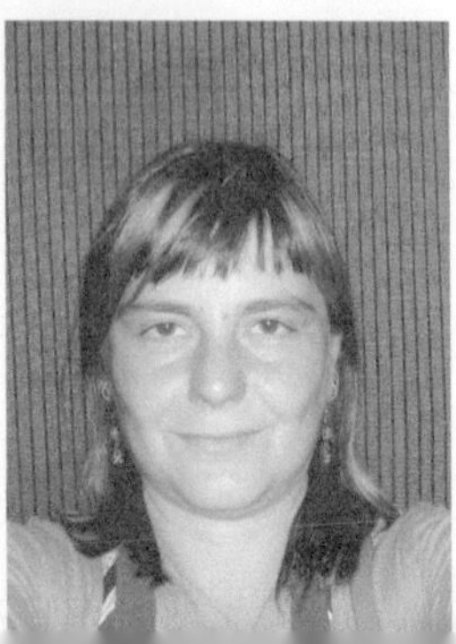

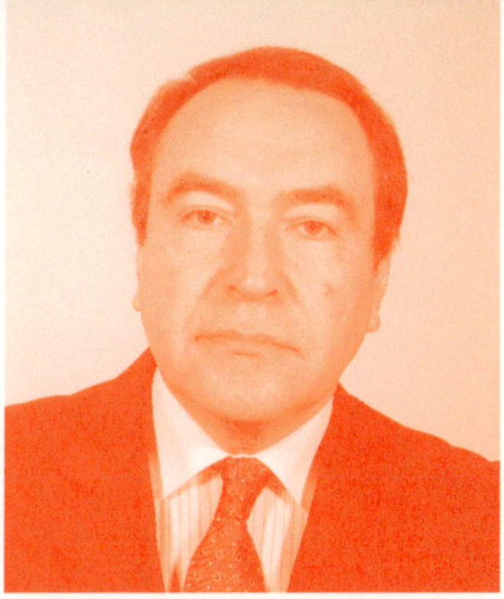
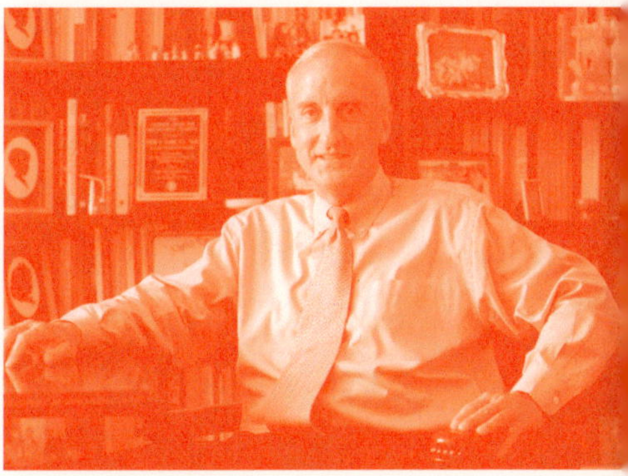
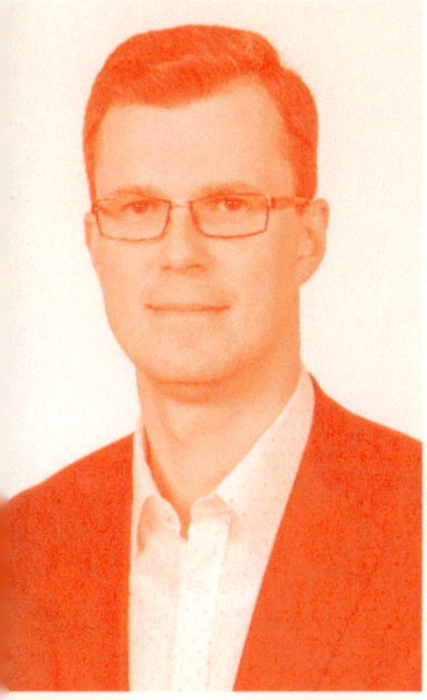
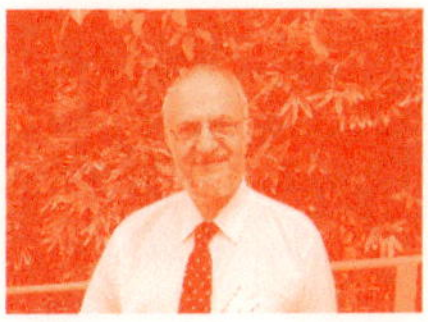
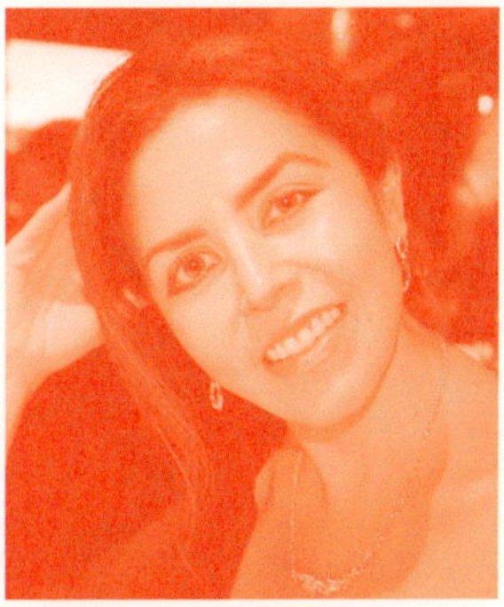

Supporting open minds since 2005

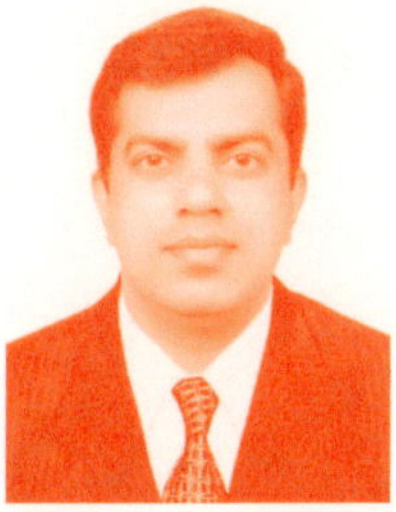
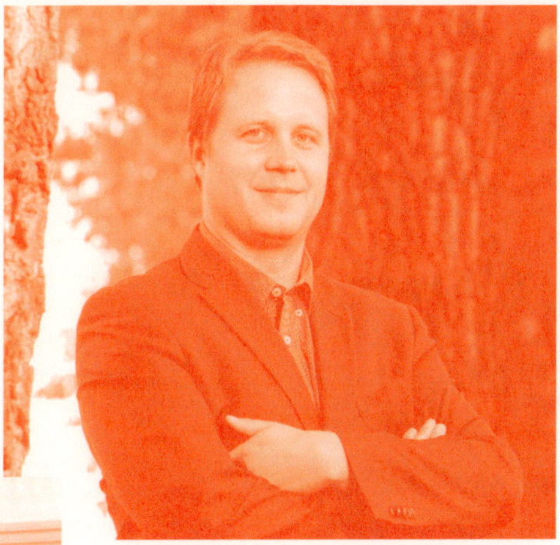
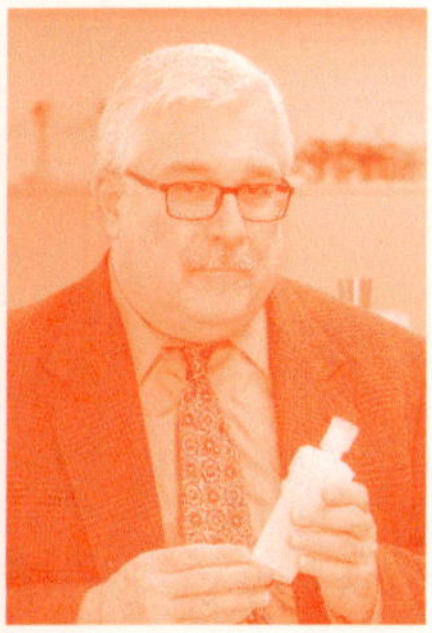
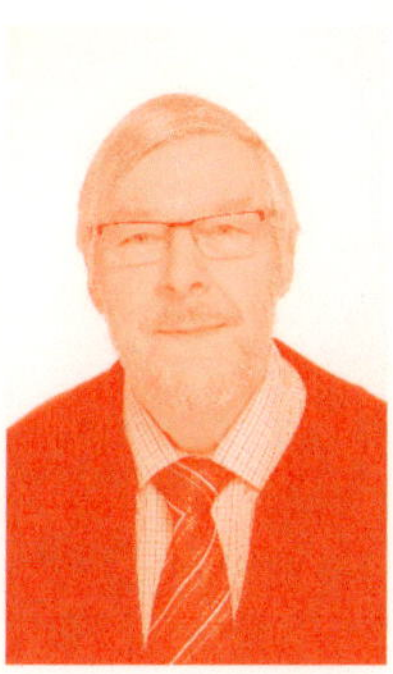
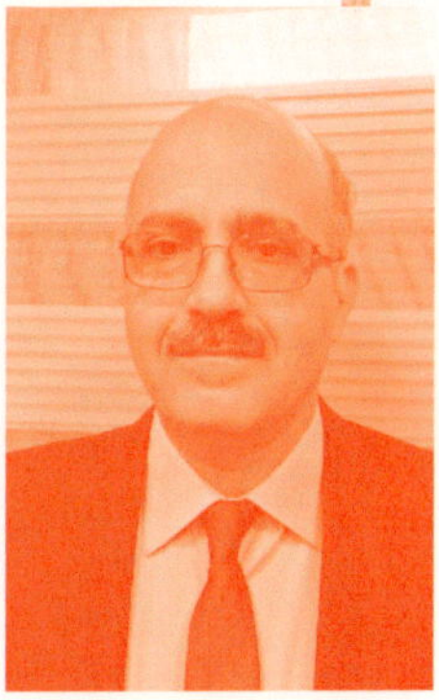
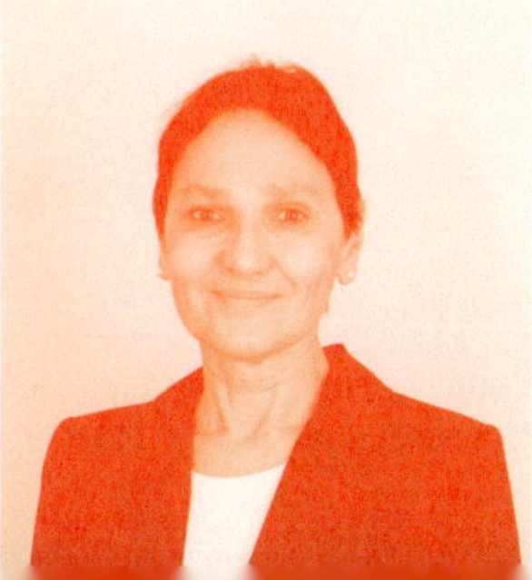
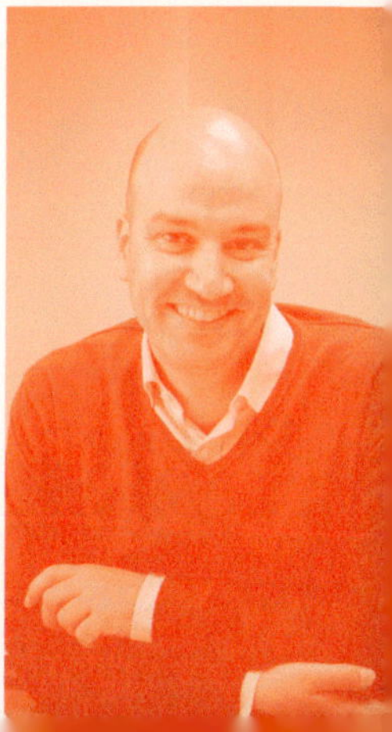

Nonalcoholic Fatty Liver Disease - An Update
http://dx.doi.org/10.5772/intechopen.78459
Edited by Emad Hamdy Gad

Contributors
Ruitang Deng, Xinmu Zhang, Ian Martins, Jibu Thomas, Subha Mary Varghese, Zaki Sherif, Diana Feier, Delia Muntean, Ahmed Ba-Ssalamah, Nina Bastati, Emad Hamdy Gad

© The Editor(s) and the Author(s) 2019
The rights of the editor(s) and the author(s) have been asserted in accordance with the Copyright, Designs and Patents Act 1988. All rights to the book as a whole are reserved by INTECHOPEN LIMITED. The book as a whole (compilation) cannot be reproduced, distributed or used for commercial or non-commercial purposes without INTECHOPEN LIMITED's written permission. Enquiries concerning the use of the book should be directed to INTECHOPEN LIMITED rights and permissions department (permissions@intechopen.com).
Violations are liable to prosecution under the governing Copyright Law.

CC BY

Individual chapters of this publication are distributed under the terms of the Creative Commons Attribution 3.0 Unported License which permits commercial use, distribution and reproduction of the individual chapters, provided the original author(s) and source publication are appropriately acknowledged. If so indicated, certain images may not be included under the Creative Commons license. In such cases users will need to obtain permission from the license holder to reproduce the material. More details and guidelines concerning content reuse and adaptation can be found at http://www.intechopen.com/copyright-policy.html.

Notice
Statements and opinions expressed in the chapters are these of the individual contributors and not necessarily those of the editors or publisher. No responsibility is accepted for the accuracy of information contained in the published chapters. The publisher assumes no responsibility for any damage or injury to persons or property arising out of the use of any materials, instructions, methods or ideas contained in the book.

First published in London, United Kingdom, 2019 by IntechOpen
IntechOpen is the global imprint of INTECHOPEN LIMITED, registered in England and Wales, registration number: 11086078, 7th floor, 10 Lower Thames Street, London, EC3R 6AF, United Kingdom
Printed in Croatia

British Library Cataloguing-in-Publication Data
A catalogue record for this book is available from the British Library

Additional hard and PDF copies can be obtained from orders@intechopen.com

Nonalcoholic Fatty Liver Disease - An Update
Edited by Emad Hamdy Gad
p. cm.
Print ISBN 978-1-83962-869-6
Online ISBN 978-1-83962-870-2
eBook (PDF) ISBN 978-1-83962-871-9

For EU product safety concerns:
IN TECH d.o.o., Prolaz Marije Krucifikse Kozulić 3, 51000 Rijeka, Croatia, info@intechopen.com or visit our website at intechopen.com.

We are IntechOpen, the world's leading publisher of Open Access books

Built by scientists, for scientists

4,400+
Open access books available

117,000+
International authors and editors

130M+
Downloads

151
Countries delivered to

Our authors are among the
Top 1%
most cited scientists

12.2%
Contributors from top 500 universities

WEB OF SCIENCE™

Selection of our books indexed in the Book Citation Index
in Web of Science™ Core Collection (BKCI)

Interested in publishing with us?
Contact book.department@intechopen.com

Numbers displayed above are based on latest data collected.
For more information visit www.intechopen.com

Meet the editor

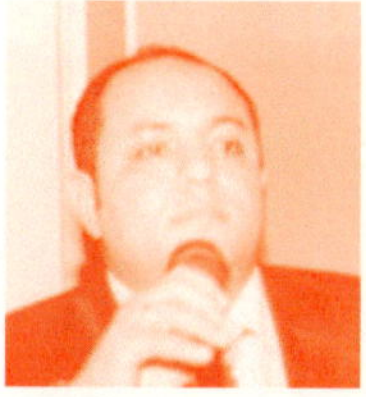

Dr. Emad Hamdy Gad is Associate Professor of Surgery in the Department of Hepatobiliary Surgery, National Liver Institute, Menoufia University, Egypt. He obtained an MD in Hepatobiliary and Liver Transplant Surgery from Menoufia University, Egypt, in 2012. Dr. Gad has published a number of research papers in reputed journals, coauthored a book chapter, and serves as a peer reviewer and editorial board member for several journals. He has also participated in international conferences as a speaker as well as a member of organizing committees.

Contents

Preface

Non-alcoholic fatty liver disease (NAFLD) is a major medical challenge because of its increasing prevalence, difficulties in diagnosis, complex pathogenesis, and lack of approved therapies. It includes a group of conditions starting with simple liver steatosis, which can develop into nonalcoholic steatohepatitis (NASH) or fibrosis, which can progress to cryptogenic cirrhosis, portal hypertension, or hepatocellular carcinoma (HCC), and finally end-stage liver failure.

In the near future, it will become the major form of chronic liver disease in adults and children and the leading indication for liver transplantation.

It can be detected by noninvasive and invasive tools, and its treatment depends mainly on lifestyle modification to prevent disease progression and its related sequelae.

Divided into four sections, this book discusses some new topics related to NAFLD. The first section provides an introduction to NAFLD, the second section presents experimental work related to the disease, the third section discusses diseases related to NAFLD, and the final section examines new noninvasive tools to diagnose NAFLD.

The book provides information on NAFLD prevalence, etiology, pathogenesis, pathology, diagnosis, and treatment as well.

Emad Hamdy Gad
Associate professor of hepatobiliary surgery,
National liver institute, Menoufia University, Egypt

Section 1

Introduction to Nonalcoholic Fatty Liver Disease

Chapter 1

Introductory Chapter: Nonalcoholic Fatty Liver Disease - What Should We Know?

Emad Hamdy Gad and Yasmin Kamel

1. Introduction

Nonalcoholic fatty liver disease (NAFLD) is considered a major challenge because of its prevalence, difficulties in diagnosis, complex pathogenesis, and lack of approved therapies. It will become the main cause of chronic liver disease in adults and children and the leading indication for liver transplantation (LT) in the next decades replacing hepatitis C virus (HCV) infection [1]. It is characterized by excessive hepatic fat accumulation, associated with insulin resistance (IR), where liver pathology shows steatosis in >5% of hepatocytes or a proton density fat fraction >5.6% assessed by proton magnetic resonance spectroscopy (1HMRS) or quantitative fat/water selective magnetic resonance imaging (MRI) [2]. It represents a group of conditions ranging from simple asymptomatic liver steatosis (nonalcoholic fatty liver (NAFL)) (known by imaging or histology) to cirrhosis (nonalcoholic steatohepatitis (NASH) or cryptogenic), end stage liver disease (ESLD), and hepatocellular carcinoma (HCC), passing through nonalcoholic steatohepatitis (NASH), which is characterized by the presence of apoptosis, ballooning, inflammation, and fibrosis with the absence of secondary causes of hepatic fat accumulation such as significant alcohol consumption or viral infection [3]. In the majority of patients, NAFLD is commonly associated with metabolic comorbidities such as obesity, type 2 DM (T2DM), and dyslipidemia. So it became common after increased prevalence of these comorbidities [4].

Our book discusses some new topics related to NAFLD, where we divided it into four sectors: the first sector includes introductory chapter about NAFLD; the second sector contains experimental work related to the disease, while the third sector discusses diseases related to NAFLD; and finally the fourth sector includes a new noninvasive tool to diagnose NAFLD. The book gives hints regarding NAFLD prevalence, etiology, pathogenesis, pathology, diagnosis, and treatment.

This introductory chapter discusses the recent updated data on the prevalence, natural history, pathophysiology, pathology, diagnosis, and treatment of the disease.

2. Natural history and disease progression

NAFLD prevalence in general population ranges between 13.48 and 31.79% differing according to diagnostic method, age, sex, and ethnicity [5, 6], while NASH prevalence in the general population ranges between 1.5 and 6.45% [5]. It is a slowly progressive disease [7]. Patients with histological NASH, especially those with some

IntechOpen

degree of fibrosis, are at higher risk for disease progression and adverse outcomes such as decompensated cirrhosis, HCC, LT, or liver-related mortality [5, 8].

3. Pathogenesis

NAFLD is tightly associated with IR not only in the liver but also in muscle and adipose tissues and also with metabolic syndrome (MetS), defined as the cluster of any three of the following five features associated with IR: impaired fasting glucose (IFG) or T2DM, hypertriglyceridemia, low high-density lipoprotein (HDL), increased waist circumference (WC), and high blood pressure. So, the presence of MetS in any given patient should lead to an evaluation of the risk of NAFLD and vice versa [9].

A high-calorie diet, saturated fats, and a high fructose intake have been associated with obesity and NAFLD [10]. It is documented that visceral obesity is one of NASH predictors; it is associated with insulin resistance, oxidative stress, inflammatory cascade, and overflow of portal triglycerides [11, 12]. So, follow-up of the disease and its progression is mandatory in obese persons.

T2DM is associated with NAFLD severity, NASH development, advanced fibrosis, and HCC [13]. It is also related to IR, obesity, dyslipedemia, and elevated liver enzymes [14].

Recently, multiple parallel hits are responsible for NAFLD pathogenesis and progression (i.e., impaired mitochondrial adenosine triphosphate (ATP) activity [15], depletion of mitochondrial glutathione [16, 17], hypoxia associated with impaired blood flow or obesity-related obstructive sleep apnea [18], dysregulated adipokine production [19], the effects of a high fructose diet [20], and rapid weight loss [21]).

However, hepatic iron is a source of oxidative stress and hepatocyte dysfunction; its role in NAFLD and NASH remains controversial [22].

Both animal and human studies support the concept that the hepatocellular injury in NAFL persons that lead to NASH is caused by overload of primary metabolic substrates (glucose, fructose, and fatty acids) in the liver, resulting in diversion of fatty acids into pathways that promote cellular injury and dysfunctional response to that injury [23, 24].

In human models and in the setting of established IR and a diet high in saturated fats, hepatic traffic of excess free fatty acids (FFA) induces hepatocyte injury via lipotoxicity, caused by oxidative stress through the generation of lipotoxic metabolites (such as ceramides, diacylglycerols, and lysophosphatidyl choline) and reactive oxygen species (ROS) [25]. However, in animal models, the oxidative stress that occurs in the setting of obesity-related IR and lipotoxicity is central to hepatocyte injury and is critical to the pathogenesis of NASH [26].

It is documented that lipotoxicity leads to hepatic cell injury and death, via apoptosis and/or necrosis, and this is an important driver of inflammation, NASH, and fibrosis [27, 28]. Oxidative stress is a major driver of hepatocyte senescence that represents a cellular stress response and an irreversible cell cycle arrest aimed to limit the proliferation of damaged cells and subsequent tumor development. Furthermore, senescent cells can mediate NAFLD progression via the active secretion of pro-inflammatory factors that affect the microenvironment, and this represents the adoption of a "senescence-associated secretory phenotype" (SASP) [26]. In NASH, the inflammatory response includes both the innate and adaptive immunity; the cascade begins with hepatocyte injury in the setting of IR and lipotoxicity and is propagated by cellular apoptosis, culminating with the activation of hepatic stellate cells (HSCs) and ensuing fibrosis [26].

In short, the pathogenesis of NASH goes as follows: Hepatocytes are affected by lifestyle factors as a high saturated fatty acid (SFA) diet, obesity, IR, and hepatic steatosis; these multiple parallel metabolic hits lead to cellular damage, via a process called "lipotoxicity," involving excessive oxidative stress principally driven by the lipotoxic metabolites of SFA. Injured hepatocytes release damage-associated metabolic patterns (DAMPs) that initiate an inflammatory response, predominantly via toll-like receptors (TLRs) and activate pro-inflammatory signaling pathways in the setting of increased adipokine levels. Furthermore, injured hepatocytes undergo necrosis, apoptosis, and senescence that have a great role in disease progression. Direct recruitment of Kupffer cells (KC) and other components of the innate immune response occurs with activation of the inflammasome and the coordinated release of pro-inflammatory and pro-fibrogenic cytokines and ligands (e.g., Hh, OPN). Also, KC promotes a pro-inflammatory microenvironment that initiates adaptive immune response. HSC are subsequently activated to produce extracellular matrix leading to progressive fibrosis, cirrhosis, and its complications (e.g., HCC). Engulfment of apoptotic bodies and factors produced by senescent cells (SASP) can also influence HSC activity directly [26].

4. Diagnosis

NAFL encompasses (a) steatosis alone; (b) steatosis with lobular or portal inflammation, without ballooning; or (c) steatosis with ballooning but without inflammation. The diagnosis of NASH requires the joint presence of steatosis, ballooning, and lobular inflammation. So, liver biopsy is essential for its diagnosis [29]. Biopsy should give comment on steatosis severity (mild, moderate, or severe). Specific scoring systems such as NAFLD activity score (NAS) and/or steatosis activity fibrosis (SAF) may be appropriate. Moreover, the presence or absence of fibrosis should be described (stage 1 is zone 3 (perivenular or perisinusoidal fibrosis) or periportal fibrosis, stage 2 is both zone 3 and periportal fibrosis, stage 3 is bridging fibrosis with nodularity, and stage 4 is cirrhosis) [5]. Because of liver biopsy invasive nature, sampling errors, cost, and its related morbidity and mortality and noninvasive tools to detect NAFL and NASH were thoroughly studied and developed. They have the following advantages: (i) identification of the risk of NAFLD in people with high metabolic risk in primary care settings, (ii) identification of those with worse prognosis (i.e., severe NASH) in secondary and tertiary care settings, and (iii) disease progression and therapeutic response monitoring [2]. US, computed tomography (CT), and MRI are noninvasive diagnostic methods of moderate and severe steatosis, and they can provide additional hepatobiliary information; hence, they should be performed as first-line diagnostic tools for steatosis [2]. Moreover, MRI, either by spectroscopy (MRS) or by proton density fat fraction (PDFF), is a good noninvasive tool for quantifying steatosis [5]; furthermore, the best-validated steatosis scores are the fatty liver index (FLI) and the SteatoTest and the NAFLD liver fat score; they variably predict metabolic, hepatic, and cardiovascular outcomes [2]. Regarding NASH, clinical, biochemical, and imaging measures cannot distinguish it from steatosis. However, cytokeratin-18 fragments (CK-18), which are generated during cell death or apoptosis, have modest accuracy for the diagnosis of NASH (66% sensitivity, 82% specificity) [5, 30]. Clinical decision aids (e.g., NAFLD fibrosis score (NFS), FIB-4 index, aspartate aminotransferase [AST] to platelet ratio index [APRI]), serum biomarkers (enhanced liver fibrosis [ELF] panel, fibrometer, FibroTest, and Hepascore), or imaging (e.g., vibration controlled transient elastography (VCTE; FibroScan), MR elastography [MRE], acoustic radiation force impulse imaging, and supersonic shear wave elastography) are acceptable noninvasive procedures for the identification of cases with advanced fibrosis or cirrhosis; furthermore, their combination might confer additional diagnostic accuracy, and monitor disease progression, saving a number of diagnostic liver biopsies [5].

5. Treatment

It is considered that NAFLD treatments are limited; as the pathogenesis of NASH (as discussed above) involves the complex interaction of cellular responses to chronic injury, furthermore, the development of the disease over many years cannot be easily repaired with short-term intervention (most updated studies have involved short-term treatment only); moreover, NAFLD is thought to be a heterogeneous disease [26]. The management of NAFLD should consist of treating liver disease as well as the associated metabolic comorbidities such as obesity, hyperlipidemia, IR, and T2DM [5].

NAFLD can be treated with lifestyle changes (i.e., healthy diet and habitual physical activity) as weight loss results in improvement of liver enzymes and histology (steatosis, hepatocyte ballooning, and necroinflammtion) and healthy diet improves IR; moreover, both aerobic exercise and resistance training reduce liver fat with no need for drug therapy if there is no NASH or fibrosis [31, 32]. However, successful treatment of NASH should improve outcomes, i.e., decrease NASH-related mortality, and reduce progression to cirrhosis or HCC [2]; this can be achieved with drug therapy that is indicated for progressive NASH (bridging fibrosis and cirrhosis), for early-stage NASH with increased risk of fibrosis progression (age > 50 years; diabetes, MetS, increased ALT) [33], and for active NASH with high necro-inflammatory activity [34].

The oxidative stress from lipotoxicity has a central role in disease progression, and therefore, the use of antioxidants and other approaches to limit this oxidative stress was considered. In some studies, vitamin E (800 IU/day) as an antioxidant improved steatosis, inflammation, and ballooning and induced resolution of NASH [35]. It may be used in non-cirrhotic nondiabetic NASH patients, but further studies are needed before making firm recommendations.

Ursodeoxycholic acid (UDCA) has been investigated in several RCTs as a treatment for NASH at different doses for up to 2 years with some biochemical improvement without any histological effect [36–38]. Recently, a negative correlation was shown between the degree of coffee intake as antioxidant and fibrosis stage in NASH. However, the role of phlebotomy in management of NASH by decreasing hepatic iron overload and its oxidative stress effect is still controversial. On the other hand and despite being under study, newer approaches for managing NASH were developed (pentoxifylline, infliximab, NK inhibitors, STAT3 blockade, and anti-CD3 therapy); they aimed at affecting the intercellular mechanisms that have a role in the pathogenesis of NASH. Also, the use of specific medical therapies that are effective in patients with metabolic comorbidities (e.g., insulin sensitizing agents (pioglitazone), statins, angiotensin-converting-enzyme inhibitors, and angiotensin-receptor blockers) has also been tried in patients with NASH with promising results [26].

Bariatric surgery decreases liver fat and NASH progression by treating obesity, IR, and diabetes; prospective data showed an improvement in histological NASH lesions, including fibrosis [39–41].

Lastly, LT is an accepted procedure in NASH patients with ESLD, liver failure, or HCC with comparable overall survival to other indications, despite a higher cardiovascular mortality [42, 43].

Finally, I think the book will give readers important knowledge regarding NAFLD.

Author details

Emad Hamdy Gad[1*] and Yasmin Kamel[2]

1 Hepatobiliary and Liver Transplantation Surgery Department, National Liver Institute, Menoufia University, Menoufia, Egypt

2 Anaesthesia Department, National Liver Institute, Menoufia University, Menoufia, Egypt

*Address all correspondence to: emadgadsalemaa@yahoo.com

IntechOpen

© 2019 The Author(s). Licensee IntechOpen. This chapter is distributed under the terms of the Creative Commons Attribution License (http://creativecommons.org/licenses/by/3.0), which permits unrestricted use, distribution, and reproduction in any medium, provided the original work is properly cited.

References

[1] Neuschwander-Tetri BA. Non-alcoholic fatty liver disease. BMC Medicine. 2017;**15**:45

[2] European Association for the Study of the Liver (EASL), European Association for the Study of Diabetes (EASD) and European Association for the Study of Obesity (EASO). EASL—EASD—EASO clinical practice guidelines for the management of non-alcoholic fatty liver disease. Journal of Hepatology. 2016;**64**:1388-1402

[3] Fierbinteanu-Braticevici C, Baicus C, Tribus L, Papacocea R. Predictive factors for nonalcoholic steatohepatitis (NASH) in patients with nonalcoholic fatty liver disease (NAFLD). Journal of Gastrointestinal and Liver Diseases. 2011;**20**(2):153-159

[4] Brunt EM, Wong VW, Nobili V, Day CP, Sookoian S, Maher JJ, et al. Nonalcoholic fatty liver disease. Nature Reviews. Disease Primers. 2015;**1**:15080

[5] Chalasani N, Younossi Z, Lavine JE, Charlton M, Cusi K, Rinella M, et al. The diagnosis and management of nonalcoholic fatty liver disease: Practice guidance from the american association for the study of liver diseases. Hepatology. 2018;**67**(1):328-357

[6] Vernon G, Baranova A, Younossi ZM. Systematic review: The epidemiology and natural history of non-alcoholic fatty liver disease and non-alcoholic steatohepatitis in adults. Alimentary Pharmacology & Therapeutics. 2011;**34**:274-228

[7] Singh S, Allen AM, Wang Z, Prokop LJ, Murad MH, Loomba R. Fibrosis progression in nonalcoholic fatty liver vs. nonalcoholic steatohepatitis: A systematic review and meta-analysis of paired-biopsy studies. Clinical Gastroenterology and Hepatology. 2015;**13**:643-654, e641–e649; quiz e639–e640

[8] Goh GB, McCullough AJ. Natural history of nonalcoholic fatty liver disease. Digestive Diseases and Sciences. 2016;**61**:1226-1233

[9] Gaggini M, Morelli M, Buzzigoli E, DeFronzo RA, Bugianesi E, Gastaldelli A. Non-alcoholic fatty liver disease (NAFLD) and its connection with insulin resistance, dyslipidemia, atherosclerosis and coronary heart disease. Nutrients. 2013;**5**:1544-1560

[10] Barrera F, George J. The role of diet and nutritional intervention for the management of patients with NAFLD. Clinics in Liver Disease. 2014;**18**:91-112

[11] Tarantino G, Saldalamacchia G, Conca P, Arena A. Non-alcoholic fatty liver disease: Further expression of the metabolic syndrome. Journal of Gastroenterology and Hepatology. 2007;**22**:293-303

[12] Jou J, Choi SS, Diehl AM. Mechanisms of disease progression in nonalcoholic fatty liver disease. Seminars in Liver Disease. 2008;**28**:370-379

[13] Loomba R, Abraham M, Unalp A, Wilson L, Lavine J, Doo E, et al. Association between diabetes, family history of diabetes, and risk of nonalcoholic steatohepatitis and fibrosis. Hepatology. 2012;**56**:943-951

[14] Ghouri N, Preiss D, Sattar N. Liver enzymes, nonalcoholic fatty liver disease, and incident cardiovascular disease: A narrative review and clinical perspective of prospective data. Hepatology. 2010;**52**:1156-1161

[15] Cortez-Pinto H, Chatham J, Chacko VP, Arnold C, Rashid A,

Diehl AM. Alterations in liver ATP homeostasis in human nonalcoholic steatohepatitis: A pilot study. JAMA. 1999;**282**:1659-1664

[16] Mari M, Caballero F, Colell A, Morales A, Caballeria J, Fernandez A, et al. Mitochondrial free cholesterol loading sensitizes to TNF- and Fas-mediated steatohepatitis. Cell Metabolism. 2006;**4**:185-198

[17] Mari M, Colell A, Morales A, Caballero F, Moles A, Fernandez A, et al. Mechanism of mitochondrial glutathione-dependent hepatocellular susceptibility to TNF despite NF-kappa B activation. Gastroenterology. 2008;**134**:1507-1520

[18] Polotsky VY, Patil SP, Savransky V, Laffan A, Fonti S, Frame LA, et al. Obstructive sleep apnea, insulin resistance, and steatohepatitis in severe obesity. American Journal of Respiratory and Critical Care Medicine. 2009;**179**:228-234

[19] Musso G, Gambino R, de Michieli F, Durazzo M, Pagano G, Cassader M. Adiponectin gene polymorphisms modulate acute adiponectin response to dietary fat: Possible pathogenetic role in NASH. Hepatology. 2008;**47**:1167-1177

[20] Abdelmalek MF, Suzuki A, Guy C, Unalp-Arida A, Colvin R, Johnson RJ, et al. Increased fructose consumption is associated with fibrosis severity in patients with nonalcoholic fatty liver disease. Hepatology. 2010;**51**:1961-1971

[21] D'Albuquerque LA, Gonzalez AM, Wahle RC, de Oliveira Souza E, Mancero JM, de Oliveira e Silva A. Liver transplantation for subacute hepatocellular failure due to massive steatohepatitis after bariatric surgery. Liver Transplantation. 2008;**14**:881-885

[22] O'Brien J, Powell LW. Non-alcoholic fatty liver disease: Is iron relevant? Hepatology International. 2012;**6**:332-341

[23] Machado MV, Diehl AM. Pathogenesis of nonalcoholic steatohepatitis. Gastroenterology. 2016;**150**:1769-1777

[24] Ertunc ME, Hotamisligil GS. Lipid signaling and lipotoxicity in metabolic inflammation: Indications for metabolic disease pathogenesis and treatment. Journal of Lipid Research. 2016;**57**:2099-2114

[25] Neuschwander-Tetri BA. Hepatic lipotoxicity and the pathogenesis of nonalcoholic steatohepatitis: The central role of nontriglyceride fatty acid metabolites. Hepatology. 2010;**52**:774-788

[26] Peverill W, Powell LW, Skoien R. Evolving concepts in the pathogenesis of NASH: Beyond steatosis and inflammation. International Journal of Molecular Sciences. 2014;**15**:8591-8638

[27] Anderson N, Borlak J. Molecular mechanisms and therapeutic targets in steatosis and steatohepatitis. Pharmacological Reviews. 2008;**60**:311-357

[28] Tetri LH, Basaranoglu M, Brunt EM, Yerian LM, Neuschwander-Tetri BA. Severe NAFLD with hepatic necroinflammatory changes in mice fed trans fats and a high-fructose corn syrup equivalent. American Journal of Physiology. Gastrointestinal and Liver Physiology. 2008;**295**:G987-G995

[29] Kleiner DE, Brunt EM. Nonalcoholic fatty liver disease: Pathologic patterns and biopsy evaluation in clinical research. Seminars in Liver Disease. 2012;**32**:3-13

[30] Kwok R, Tse YK, Wong GL, Ha Y, Lee AU, Ngu MC, et al. Systematic review with meta-analysis: Non-invasive assessment of non-alcoholic

fatty liver disease–the role of transient elastography and plasma cytokeratin-18 fragments. Alimentary Pharmacology & Therapeutics. 2014;**39**:254-269

[31] Zelber-Sagi S, Godos J, Salomone F. Lifestyle changes for the treatment of nonalcoholic fatty liver disease: A review of observational studies and intervention trials. Therapeutic Advances in Gastroenterology. 2016;**9**:392-407

[32] Orci LA, Gariani K, Oldani G, Delaune V, Morel P, Toso C. Exercise-based interventions for nonalcoholic fatty liver disease: A meta-analysis and meta-regression. Clinical Gastroenterology and Hepatology. 2016;**14**:1398-1411

[33] Adams LA, Sanderson S, Lindor KD, Angulo P. The histological course of nonalcoholic fatty liver disease: A longitudinal study of 103 patients with sequential liver biopsies. Journal of Hepatology. 2005;**42**:132-138

[34] Sanyal AJ, Friedman SL, McCullough AJ, Dimick-Santos L. Challenges and opportunities in drug and biomarker development for nonalcoholic steatohepatitis: Findings and recommendations from an American Association for the Study of Liver Diseases-U.S. Food and Drug Administration joint workshop. Hepatology. 2015;**61**:1392-1405

[35] Sanyal AJ, Chalasani N, Kowdley KV, McCullough A, Diehl AM, Bass NM, et al. Pioglitazone, vitamin E, or placebo for nonalcoholic steatohepatitis. The New England Journal of Medicine. 2010;**362**:1675-1685

[36] Lindor KD, Kowdley KV, Heathcote EJ, Harrison ME, Jorgensen R, Angulo P, et al. Ursodeoxycholic acid for treatment of nonalcoholic steatohepatitis: Results of a randomized trial. Hepatology. 2004;**39**:770-778

[37] Dufour JF, Oneta CM, Gonvers JJ, Bihl F, Cerny A, Cereda JM, et al. Randomized placebo-controlled trial of ursodeoxycholic acid with vitamin E in nonalcoholic steatohepatitis. Clinical Gastroenterology and Hepatology. 2006;**4**:1537-1543

[38] Leuschner UF, Lindenthal B, Herrmann G, Arnold JC, Rossle M, Cordes HJ, et al. High-dose ursodeoxycholic acid therapy for nonalcoholic steatohepatitis: A double-blind, randomized, placebo-controlled trial. Hepatology. 2010;**52**:472-479

[39] Schauer PR, Bhatt DL, Kirwan JP, Wolski K, Brethauer SA, Navaneethan SD, et al. Bariatric surgery versus intensive medical therapy for diabetes. 3-Year outcomes. The New England Journal of Medicine. 2014;**370**:2002-2013

[40] Caiazzo R, Lassailly G, Leteurtre E, Baud G, Verkindt H, Raverdy V, et al. Roux-en-Y gastric bypass versus adjustable gastric banding to reduce nonalcoholic fatty liver disease: A 5-year controlled longitudinal study. Annals of Surgery. 2014;**260**:893-898

[41] Lassailly G, Caiazzo R, Buob D, Pigeyre M, Verkindt H, Labreuche J, et al. Bariatric surgery reduces features of non-alcoholic steatohepatitis in morbidly obese patients. Gastroenterology. 2015;**149**:377-388

[42] Charlton MR, Burns JM, Pedersen RA, Watt KD, Heimbach JK, Dierkhising RA. Frequency and outcomes of liver transplantation for nonalcoholic steatohepatitis in the United States. Gastroenterology. 2011;**141**:1249-1253

[43] Wang X, Li J, Riaz DR, Shi G, Liu C, Dai Y. Outcomes of liver transplantation for nonalcoholic steatohepatitis: A systematic review and meta-analysis. Clinical Gastroenterology and Hepatology. 2014;**12**:e391

Section 2

Experimental Work

Chapter 2

The Effect of *M. latifolia* Leaf Extract on High-Fructose Corn Syrup (HFCS)-Induced Non-alcoholic Fatty Liver Disease in Rat Models

Subha Mary Varghese and Jibu Thomas

Abstract

Non-alcoholic fatty liver disease (NAFLD) is a condition where the content of intrahepatic triglycerides (steatosis) rises, inclusive or exclusive of inflammation and fibrosis (namely steatohepatitis). It is acknowledged all over the world as the leading cause of chronic liver disease (CLD). Mulberry, a phytonutrient-rich plant belongs to the genus *Morus*, has been widely used as one of the conventional medicinal plants due to its chemical composition and pharmacological utility. Identification of leaf extract (*M. latifolia*) revealed chlorogenic acid, rutin, quercetin, caffeic acid and coumaric acid as functional bioactive principles. Objective of the current study was to evaluate the beneficial effect of *M. latifolia* in treating HFCS-induced metabolic disorders, namely, dyslipidaemia and non-alcoholic fatty liver disease (NAFLD), in rat models. Study determined body weight, blood glucose, lipid profile, liver marker enzymes and histopathology of liver tissues. Study concluded that administration of *M. latifolia* leaf extract showed a significant decrease in body weight and the levels of lipid profile, blood glucose and liver marker enzymes in HFCS-induced rats compared to HFCS control rats. Histopathological studies confirmed the antihyperlipidaemic properties of *M. latifolia* leaf extract in reducing the hepatic fat accumulation causing regeneration of liver tissues in HFCS-fed rats.

Keywords: HFCS, NAFLD, mulberry leaf, dyslipidaemia

1. Introduction

Obesity has become a major public health problem worldwide and is of crucial concern in the field of preventive medicine. It is a medical condition where excessive lipid is accumulated in the body, which results in increased adipose tissue mass and dysregulation of lipid metabolism. The prevalence of obesity has rapidly increased in the past few decades due to changes in lifestyle factors, especially diet [1]. Obesity is closely associated with diseases such as non-alcoholic fatty liver disease (NAFLD), hypertension, hyperlipidaemia, arteriosclerosis and cancer [1–3].

IntechOpen

Non-alcoholic fatty liver disease (NAFLD) results in a rise in content of intrahepatic triglyceride (IHTG) (i.e. steatosis), inclusive or exclusive of inflammation and fibrosis (namely steatohepatitis). Today, NAFLD is acknowledged all over the world as the leading cause of chronic liver disease (CLD). The condition brings about an extreme accretion of hepatocytes. It comprises a pathological field varying from mild, harmless steatosis to acute, critical non-alcoholic steatohepatitis, liver fibrosis, cirrhosis and hepatocellular carcinoma (HCC) [4]. NAFLD is generally linked to insulin resistance and considered as the hepatic expression of the metabolic disorder. There is a great dearth of pharmacological remedies presently for the treatment of NAFLD, with intentional changes in lifestyle such as weight loss through wholesome diet and exercise the only known means for bringing about an improvement in the status.

A predominant factor behind the sudden escalation of obesity is the use of high-fructose corn syrup in beverages. It is found that HFCS embodies >40% of caloric sweeteners which are included in foods and beverages. Furthermore, it is the primary caloric sweetener added in soft drinks in the USA, where the cases of obesity are steadily rising as a result. The drawback of HFCS is that the digestion, absorption and metabolism of fructose vary from that of glucose. Hepatic metabolism of fructose supports de novo lipogenesis. Moreover, fructose does not promote the secretion of insulin or improvement of leptin generation. As insulin and leptin serve as crucial afferent signals in the control of food consumption and body weight, it indicates that dietary fructose may be instrumental in enlarged energy intake and a rise in weight. Additionally, calorically sweetened beverages are likely to intensify caloric consumption. These given factors suggest that the heightened ingestion of HFCS and its excessive intake through various liquid refreshments are decisive in the surge of obesity in recent times [5].

Current findings show HFCS-55 consumption to modify hepatic lipid metabolism and increase the amassment of triglycerides. HFCS-55 is considered to be more lipogenic than sucrose, which greatly raises the danger of developing non-alcoholic fatty liver disease (NAFLD) and dyslipidaemia. Rats which imbibed HFCS-55 solution were found to have the highest ($P = .03$) hepatic total lipid and triglyceride content as well as histological evidence for fat penetration [6].

Natural bioactive substances contained in fruits and vegetables inclusive of phenolic compounds, flavonoids and anthocyanins have generated widespread interest owing to their antioxidant properties. They are being steadily looked upon as possible remedies to combat obesity and obesity-related metabolic syndrome [7–10].

Mulberry is a phytonutrient-rich plant which belongs to the genus *Morus* and family Moraceae. It has been widely used as one of the conventional medicinal plants for centuries due to its chemical composition and pharmacological utility [11]. Mulberry leaves can be regarded as potential sources of phytochemical compounds with verified biological properties. The latest reports suggest mulberry leaves (*Morus alba* L.) to be a rich source of polyphenolic substances, including phenolic acids and flavonoids [12]. Earlier studies have revealed mulberry leaves to possess anticholesteremic effects [13] and cardiovascular and hepatoprotective properties [14, 15]. In more recent past, Song et al. [4] evaluated the positive impact of mulberry fruit extract on NAFLD present in mice fed on a high-fat diet.

The main objective of the current study is to evaluate the beneficial effect of *Morus latifolia* leaf extract in treating HFCS-induced metabolic disorders, namely, dyslipidaemia and non-alcoholic fatty liver disease (NAFLD), in rat models.

2. Materials and methods

2.1 Collection of plant material

Twigs of *M. latifolia* var. BC 259 were collected from the germplasm collections of Sericulture Department, Tamil Nadu Agricultural University, Coimbatore. Five to seven leaves from the apex were plucked and shade dried.

2.2 Preparation of *M. latifolia* leaf extract

Mulberry leaves of BC 259 were dried overnight at 90°C, and 20 g was powdered and extracted with 70% ethanol using the Soxhlet apparatus. The extract obtained was further separated with chloroform and ethyl acetate using a separating funnel. The polyphenolic ethyl acetate layer finally acquired was evaporated using rotary evaporator and was taken for its quantification of polyphenolic constituent profile using HPLC [16].

2.3 Identification of polyphenolic compounds by HPLC and its quantification

Phenolic constituents were determined using the HPLC method described by Rodriguez et al. [17]. Chromatographic conditions include separation in HPLC (Waters, Model: 515) fitted with photodiode array detector (Model: 2998) and ODS column (250 mm × 4.6 mm, 4 μm) (Hichrom, USA). Binary elution was performed with solvents (methanol-acetic acid-water) in the proportion of 10:2:88 and 90:2:8 as mobile phases A and B, respectively. Measurements were made at 254 and 280 nm. Phenolic acids were identified based on the retention time and UV spectrum of reference standards. Reference standards at concentrations (10–40 μg/mL) were injected into the HPLC-DAD system, and the calibration curves were generated. Concentrations of the compounds were calculated from peak area according to the generated calibration curves.

2.4 Animals

Animal studies were performed with 30 male Wistar rats weighing ~200 g procured from Veterinary College, Thrissur, Kerala. Animals were acclimatized at a temperature of 25 ± 2°C with a relative humidity of 45–55% in a 12-hour light-dark cycle and were fed with standard laboratory diet (rat chow diet) where water was given ad libitum. Rats used in the study were maintained in accordance with guidelines of the Institutional Animal Ethical Committee of the University. Institutional Animal Ethical Committee's (IAEC) approval was obtained under experiment no. IAEC/KU/BT/13/02 for the present study.

2.5 Experimental design

Rats were divided into five groups with six rats each, and they were treated as follows: Group I, normal control rats (non-obesity control); Group II, high-fructose corn syrup (HFCS 20%)-induced obese rats; Group III, obese rats with standard drug, orlistat (120 mg/kg body weight); Group IV, obese rats with *Morus latifolia* leaf extract at dose of 250 mg/kg/day; and Group V, obese rats with *Morus latifolia* leaf extract at dose of 500 mg/kg/day. The treatment was continued orally for 21 days (3 weeks).

2.6 Experimental induction of obesity

All rats (four groups) except normal group were fed with HFCS (G55) dissolved in water to a final concentration of 20% through liquid diet in a feeding bottle with a capacity of 125 mL to achieve obesity, while normal control rats were fed with water. This diet was fed to rats of Group II to Group V for 21 days from the start of experiment. The obese rats (Group III) were treated with standard drug orlistat (200 mg/kg), and Groups IV and V were treated with *Morus latifolia* (BC 259) leaf extract with water at doses 250 and 500 mg/kg/day, respectively, for 21 days. The dosages were administered orally using an oral gavage.

2.7 Body weight

The body weight of the experimental animals was recorded prior to treatment and before sacrificing the animals according to the experimental schedule.

2.8 Biochemical analysis

At the end of the experimental period (21 days), after euthanizing the animals, the blood was withdrawn by cardiac puncture, and the blood samples were centrifuged (10,000 rpm/10 min at room temperature) to get the serum. The serum was transferred into the Eppendorf tubes to be stored at −20°C.

The serum collected during the post-treatment periods were analyzed with commercially available assay kits (ERBA Diagnostics, Mannheim, Germany) for determination of the levels of glucose (glucose oxidase/peroxidase (GOD/POD) method), lipid profile levels for high-density lipoprotein cholesterol (HDL-C), total cholesterol (TC) and triglycerides (TG).

LDL-C was calculated using Friedewald's equation [18]:

$$\text{LDL} - \text{C} = [\text{TC} - \{\text{HDL} + (\text{TG}/5)\}]. \quad (1)$$

VLDL-C levels were calculated by subtracting the sum of HDL-C and LDL-C concentrations from TC [19].

Liver marker enzymes such as aspartate aminotransferase (AST), alanine aminotransferase (ALT) and alkaline phosphatase (ALP) present in serum were also estimated with assay kits (ERBA Diagnostics, Mannheim, Germany). After the animals were euthanized by ether overdose, they were sacrificed by cervical dislocation.

2.9 Histopathology of liver tissue

The liver was dissected and washed with ice-cold saline immediately to remove the blood. The liver was immediately transferred to the fixative of 10% formalin. The tissues were dehydrated and embedded in paraffin wax to make it firm for section cutting. A section of 6 μm was made and stained in hematoxylin and eosin dye for microscopic observations [20].

2.10 Data analysis

Data generated was presented as mean value ± standard error mean (SEM) for all experimental groups. Statistical analysis was performed using SPSS version 16.0 to conduct one-way analysis of variance (ANOVA) followed by Duncan's Multiple Range test (DMRT) to find out the significant differences among the various treatment groups wherever possible. Values corresponding to $p < 0.05$ were considered statistically significant.

3. Results

3.1 Effect of *M. latifolia* (var. BC 259) leaf extract on serum glucose level in HFCS-fed rats

Table 1 represents the effect of *M. latifolia* leaf extract on changes in serum glucose level in HFCS-fed rats. In HFCS-fed rats, there was a significant increase in blood glucose level (178.14 mg/dL) compared to normal control rats (89.83 mg/dL). On the other hand, HFCS-fed rats treated with standard orlistat reduced the blood glucose level to an extent of 111.87 mg/dL compared to HFCS control group ($p < 0.05$). Both the concentrations of *M. latifolia* leaf extract kept the glucose level under control compared to HFCS control group (HFCS 20%) at $p < 0.01$. The degree of reduction of the blood glucose by standard drug and *M. latifolia* leaf extract at 500 mg/kg was statistically the same.

3.2 Effect of *M. latifolia* leaf extract on body weight in HFCS-fed rats

The effect of *M. latifolia* leaf extract on body weight in HFCS-fed rats is represented in **Table 2**. Normal control rats registered 182.20 g body weight at the end of the experimental period. Contrary to normal control rats, HFCS-fed rats showed drastic increase in body weight (280.74 g) compared to normal control rats. HFCS-fed rats treated with standard drug reduced the body weight by 31.54% compared to HFCS control rats. Oral administration of *M. latifolia* leaf extract at 250 and 500 mg/kg body weight reduced the body weight significantly at $p < 0.05$ compared to HFCS control rats. The percentage of decrease in body weight was 25 and 29%, respectively.

3.3 Effect of *M. latifolia* leaf extract on lipid profile in HFCS-fed rats

The serum lipid profiles of rats at the end of the experiments are illustrated in **Table 3**. Untreated HFCS-fed rats had enhanced levels of total cholesterol and triglycerides and decreased levels of HDL compared to normal control rats. A significant reduction in the levels of serum cholesterol and triglycerides was observed in HFCS-induced rats on administration with standard drug orlistat (200 mg/kg) or mulberry leaf extract at 250 or 500 mg/kg compared with HFCS control rats ($p < 0.05$). It may be noted that the effect of standard drug and *M. latifolia* leaf extract at 500 mg/kg was found to be statistically the same based on DMRT. A

Groups	Glucose (mg/dL)
Normal control rats	89.83 ± 5.91^{a}
HFCS control rats	178.14 ± 11.82^{d}
HFCS + orlistat (120 mg/kg)	111.87 ± 7.37^{b}
MLE (250 mg/kg) + HFCS (20%)	139.45 ± 9.23^{c}
MLE (500 mg/kg) + HFCS (20%)	116.43 ± 7.70^{b}

n = 6 in each group; values were presented as mean ± standard deviation. The superscript letters $^{a–d}$ in the column represent significant difference between each treatment group at 5% probability.

Table 1.
Effect of M. latifolia leaf extract on serum glucose level in HFCS-fed rats.

Groups	Final body weight (g)
Normal control rats	182.20 ± 11.06[a]
HFCS (20%) control rats	280.74 ± 16.60[d]
HFCS + orlistat (120 mg/kg)	192.17 ± 11.29[a,b]
MLE (250 mg/kg) + HFCS (20%)	210.54 ± 12.19[c]
MLE (500 mg/kg) + HFCS (20%)	198.37 ± 11.06[b,c]

n = 6 in each group; values presented are mean ± standard deviation. The superscript letters [a–d] in the column represent significant difference between each treatment group at 5% probability.

Table 2.
Effect of M. latifolia leaf extract on body weight in HFCS-fed rats.

Groups	TC (mg/dl)	TG (mg/dl)	HDL (mg/dl)	LDL (mg/dl)	VLDL (mg/dl)
Normal control rats	142.45 ± 8.85[a]	80.29 ± 4.42[a]	55.70 ± 3.32[d]	71.79 ± 4.20[a]	16.05 ± 0.97[a]
HFCS (20%) control rats	268.57 ± 16.60[c]	182.45 ± 10.89[c]	24.14 ± 1.38[a]	207.94 ± 12.30[c]	36.49 ± 2.21[c]
HFCS + orlistat (120 mg/kg)	148.45 ± 8.85[a]	82.10 ± 3.32[a]	53.70 ± 3.15[cd]	78.33 ± 4.64 a,b	16.42 ± 1.02[a]
MLE (250 mg/kg) + HFCS (20%)	172.85 ± 10.31[b]	116.21 ± 6.96[b]	42.34 ± 2.43[b]	84.11.11 ± 5.01[b]	23.20 ± 1.46[b]
MLE (500 mg/kg) + HFCS (20%)	150.38 ± 9.05[a]	85.47 ± 5.09[a]	51.90 ± 3.05[c]	81.39 ± 4.87[b]	17.09 ± 1.04[a]

n = 6 in each group; values presented are mean ± standard deviation. The superscript letters [a–d] in the column represent significant difference between each treatment group at 5% probability.
TC, total cholesterol; TG, triglycerides; HDL, high-density lipoprotein; LDL, low-density lipoprotein; VLDL, very-low-density lipoprotein.

Table 3.
Effect of M. latifolia (var. BC 259) leaf extract on levels of serum TC, TG, HDL, LDL and VLDL in normal and HFCS-fed rats.

Groups	ALT (U/dL)	AST (U/dL)	ALP (U/dL)
Normal control rats	35.45 ± 2.01[a]	49.54 ± 2.89[a]	101.94 ± 5.98[a]
HFCS (20%) control rats	56.77 ± 3.31[e]	112.31 ± 6.63[e]	192.76 ± 11.36[d]
HFCS + orlistat (120 mg/kg)	38.43 ± 2.24[b]	61 ± 3.6[b]	124.56 ± 7.34[b]
MLE (250 mg/kg) + HFCS (20%)	51.31 ± 3.01[d]	75 ± 4.44[c]	152.31 ± 9.00[c]
MLE (500 mg/kg) + HFCS (20%)	42.15 ± 2.48[c]	63 ± 3.73[b]	132.31 ± 7.81[b]

n = 6 in each group; values presented are mean ± standard deviation. The superscript letters [a–d] in the column represent significant difference between each treatment group at 5% probability.
AST, aspartate transaminase; ALT, alanine transaminase; ALP, alkaline phosphatase.

Table 4.
Effect of M. latifolia leaf extract on levels of liver marker enzymes in HFCS-fed rats.

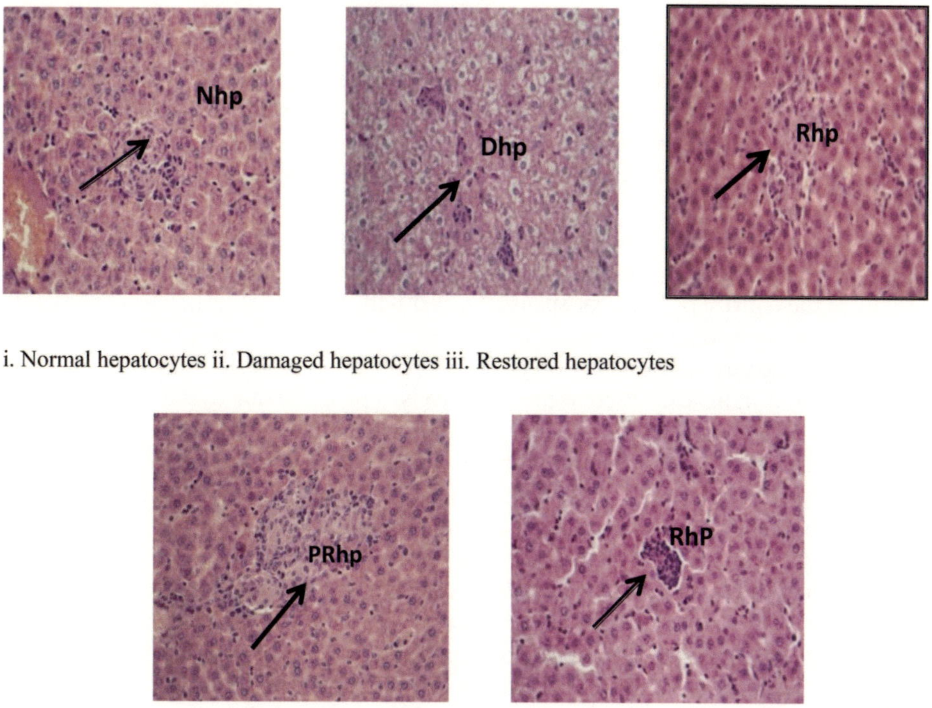

i. Normal hepatocytes ii. Damaged hepatocytes iii. Restored hepatocytes

iv. Partially recovered hepatocytes v. Recovered hepatocytes

Figure 1.
(i–v) Histopathology of the fatty liver changes in HFCS-fed rats after treatment with M. latifolia leaf extract. (i) Photomicrographs of liver tissues of untreated control rats showing normal hepatocytes. (ii) HFCS-fed rats show distorted architecture with severe fatty liver changes. (iii) Orlistat-treated rats show complete restoration of liver tissues with normal hepatocytes. (iv) M. latifolia (250 mg/kg)-treated rats show partial restoration of liver tissues with moderate fatty liver changes. (v) M. latifolia (500 mg/kg)-treated rats show maximal restoration of liver tissues with minimal fatty liver changes. Magnification at 40×.

significant improvement in HDL cholesterol was noticed in rats treated with standard drug or rats treated with mulberry leaf extract at 250 or 500 mg/kg.

3.4 Effect of *M. latifolia* leaf extract on levels of liver marker enzymes

Normal control rats registered values of 35.45 U/dL for ALT, 49.54 U/dL for AST and 101.94 U/dL for ALP (**Table 4**). Untreated HFCS-fed rats showed significantly increased levels of these enzymes compared to normal control rats ($p < 0.05$). When the test animals were treated either with orlistat or mulberry leaf extract at 250 or 500 mg/kg, there was a significant reduction in the production of ALT, AST and ALP levels.

3.5 Histopathological evaluation of liver treated with *M. latifolia* leaf extract

Photomicrographs of liver tissues of normal control rats and HFCS-fed rats after treatment with *M. latifolia* are depicted in **Figure 1(i–v)**.

4. Discussion

The consumption of fructose has seen a huge surge in the last few years, specifically in its fundamental form, high-fructose corn syrup (HFCS, 10–53%

glucose and 42–90% fructose). HFCS is utilized as a sweetener in processed foods, baked goods, condiments, soft drinks, candy, dairy products and concentrated fruit juices. It is seen to be a key factor in various diseases afflicting mankind, such as obesity, diabetes and cancer [21]. HFCS (55), which comprises 55% fructose and 45% glucose, is considered to be more lipogenic than sucrose, thus posing a great risk in the development of non-alcoholic fatty liver disease (NAFLD) and dyslipidaemia.

In contrast to glucose, fructose does not facilitate the secretion of insulin or improvement of leptin generation. As insulin and leptin serve as crucial afferent signals in the control of food consumption and body weight, it indicates that dietary fructose may be instrumental in enlarged energy intake and a rise in weight [5]. In the present study, administration of HFCS effectively induced obesity in rats as evidenced by a significant increase in body weight possibly due to the mechanism mentioned above. Supplementation of mulberry leaf extract showed a tendency towards reduction of body weight caused by HFCS. Bocarsly and his co-workers [22] reported an increase in the body weight of rats consuming HFCS, and their results coincide with data obtained in the present study.

The metabolism of fructose in the liver results in the formation of circulating triglyceride in the blood stream which will eventually lead to insulin resistance and hyperglycaemia. In the present study, HFCS has increased the serum glucose level by the stated mechanism. The administration of *Morus latifolia* leaf extract decreased the serum glucose due to the positive effect of polyphenolic extract of mulberry on glucose homoeostasis. Song et al. [4] suggested that mulberry fruit ethanol extract administration significantly improved insulin sensitivity in high-fat-fed mice.

In the present endeavor, the levels of triglycerides and total cholesterol were enhanced in HFCS-fed rats compared to normal control rats. The data obtained from the current study indicated that the model was successful in inducing hyperlipidaemia in rats. The latest findings show HFCS-55 intake to adversely affect hepatic lipid metabolism and increase the build-up of triglycerides [6]. Over the experimental period, treatment with *M. latifolia* leaf extract ameliorated the abnormalities in lipid profile as indicated by the significant ($p < 0.05$) decrease in serum triglycerides, cholesterol and LDL in HFCS-fed rats compared with untreated HFCS control rats. The degree of decrease of TC and TG levels and LDL induced by mulberry leaf extract (500 mg/kg body weight) suggested that mulberry leaf extract had a potent lipid lowering effect in hyperlipidaemia rats. Compared to normal control group, there was a significant decrease in HDL in HFCS control rats. In this study, we found that administration of *M. latifolia* leaf extract raised HDL levels in HFCS-fed animals. This rise in HDL may be the result of antiobesity effect caused by the inhibition of dyslipidaemia, hepatosteatosis and oxidative stress in obese rats [23, 24].

Yang et al. [25] found that administration of freeze-dried mulberry fruit powder resulted in a significant decrease in the serum levels of TC, TG and LDL and the hepatic levels of TG and TC and an increase in HDL in high-fat-fed rats. Chang et al. [26] illustrated from their studies that mulberry leaf polyphenol extract (MLPE) improves obesity by inducing adipocyte apoptosis and inhibiting pre-adipocyte differentiation and hepatic lipogenesis. They found quercetin and caffeic acids to be the main ingredients of MLPE which inhibit the differentiation of 3T3-L1 pre-adipocytes. Orally administering MLPE significantly reduced body weight gain and lipid accumulation in the liver and serum/hepatic triglyceride and total cholesterol levels compared with those in high-fat diet (HFD) group. Song et al. [4] demonstrated the effect of ethanolic extract of mulberry fruit in reducing HFD-induced obesity and hepatic steatosis in mice.

The protective effect of mulberry ethanol extract was associated with the induction of fatty acid oxidation and decreased fatty acid and cholesterol biosynthesis. Our results are also at par? with Andallu et al. [27]. Results obtained from the present study substantiated the earlier findings as well [13, 28, 29].

From the current study, the major polyphenolic compounds identified in *M. latifolia* were chlorogenic acid, caffeic acid, coumaric acid, rutin and quercetin. Studies have indicated that rutin could significantly reduce the levels of oleic acid-induced lipid accumulation through reducing lipogenesis and oxidative stress in hepatic carcinoma cells [30]. Previous studies have also shown that rutin may possess antiobesity effects in decreasing body weight, improving serum lipid profiles and regulating lipid metabolism [31]. Similarly, quercetin has been reported to have antiobesity effects in promoting hepatic lipolysis [32], inhibiting adipocyte differentiation, suppressing adipocytes adipogenesis, decreasing body weight [33] and improving serum lipid profiles [28]. Taher et al. [34] reported that caffeic acid isolated from *Arctium lappa* has antihyperlipidaemic effect in hyperlipidaemic rat models. Caffeic acid was reported to have antiobesity effects in decreasing body weight [35], attenuating fatty liver [36], promoting hepatic lipolysis [37] and regulating lipid metabolism [35].

Antihyperlipidaemic activity of p-coumaric acid in diabetic rats was also reported [38]. Based on these reports, we infer that crude plant extract contributing to the antiobesity effect would be due to the multiple bioactive polyphenolic compounds present in *M. latifolia* which had played a major beneficial role in treating the abnormalities in lipid metabolism.

In the present study, the increased level of liver marker enzymes (AST, ALT and ALP) was reduced and attained near-normal values when the animal groups were administrated with mulberry leaf extract. Similar results were obtained by Song and his co-workers [4] who reported that serum ALT and AST levels were reduced when the rats were fed with mulberry leaf ethanolic extract. High-fructose diets have induced fatty liver in rats [39]. NAFLD is characterized by lipid deposition in the liver, that is, steatosis [40]. Meli et al. [41] established that HFD induced hepatic steatosis in mice and rats. In addition, Chien et al. [42] reported that HFD feeding significantly increased liver weight, hepatic triglycerides and total cholesterol accumulation and hepatic vacuoles.

In this study, histological analysis of livers revealed that mulberry leaf extract administration reduced attenuated hepatic fat accumulation, even causing a regeneration of liver tissues. This has also been corroborated with reduced triglycerides and total cholesterols and serum ALT and AST levels in the mulberry leaf extract administrated group of rats. Identical results were reported earlier by Song et al. [4] with special reference to histopathological studies.

In conclusion, the results established that mulberry leaf extract amelioration improved hepatic steatosis which is due to lowered serum TC and TG levels. The study further suggested that mulberry leaf extract could be a natural dietary choice in the management of metabolic disorders such as obesity and fatty liver disease probably due to the presence of bioactive constituents, and it provides valuable input in adding to the current knowledge of the human nutrition and health.

Author details

Subha Mary Varghese and Jibu Thomas*
Department of Biotechnology, School of Agriculture and Biosciences, Karunya Institute of Technology and Sciences, Coimbatore, Tamilnadu, India

*Address all correspondence to: jibuthomas.t@gmail.com

IntechOpen

© 2019 The Author(s). Licensee IntechOpen. This chapter is distributed under the terms of the Creative Commons Attribution License (http://creativecommons.org/licenses/by/3.0), which permits unrestricted use, distribution, and reproduction in any medium, provided the original work is properly cited.

References

[1] Kopelman PG. Obesity as a medical problem. Nature. 2000;**404**:635-643

[2] Tilg H, Moschen AR. Evolution of inflammation in non-alcoholic fatty liver disease: The multiple parallel hits hypothesis. Hepatology. 2010;**52**(5):1836-1846

[3] Wellen KE, Hotamisligil GS. Inflammation, stress and diabetes. Journal of Clinical Investigation. 2005;**115**:1111-1119

[4] Song H, Lai J, Tang Q, Zheng X. Mulberry ethanol extract attenuates hepatic steatosis and insulin resistance in high-fat diet-fed mice. Nutrition Research. 2016;**36**(7):710-718

[5] Bray GA, Nielsen SJ, Popkin BM. Consumption of high-fructose corn syrup in beverages may play a role in the epidemic of obesity. The American Journal of Clinical Nutrition. 2004;**79**(4):537-543

[6] Mock K, Lateef S, Benedito VA, Tou JC. High-fructose corn syrup-55 consumption alters hepatic lipid metabolism and promotes triglyceride accumulation. The Journal of Nutritional Biochemistry. 2017;**39**:32-39

[7] Valenti L, Riso P, Mazzocchi A, Porrini M, Fargion S, Agostini C. Dietary anthocyanins as nutritional therapy for nonalcoholic fatty liver disease. Oxidative Medicine and Cellular Longevity. 2013;**2013**:145421

[8] Gossard AA, Lindor KD. Current therapies for nonalcoholic fatty liver disease. Drug Today. 2011;**47**:915-922

[9] Dembinska-Kiec A, Mykkanen O, Kiec-Wilk B, Mykkanen H. Antioxidant phytochemicals against type 2 diabetes. British Journal of Nutrition. 2008;**99E**(Suppl. 1):ES109-ES117

[10] Wang S, Moustaid-Moussa N, Chen L, Mo H, Shastri A, Su R, et al. Novel insights of dietary polyphenols and obesity. Journal of Nutritional Biochemistry. 2014;**25**:1-18

[11] Ramesh HL, Sivaram V, Murthy VNY. Antioxidant and medicinal properties of mulberry. World Journal of Pharmaceutical Research. 2014;**3**(6):320-343

[12] Memon AA, Memon N, Luthria DL, Bhanger MI, Pitafi AA. Phenolic acids profiling and antioxidant potential of Mulberry (*Morus laevigata* W., *Morus nigra* L., *Morus alba* L.) leaves and fruits grown in Pakistan. Polish Journal of Food and Nutrition Sciences. 2010;**60**(1):25-32

[13] Chan KC, Yang MY, Lin MC, Lee YJ, Chang WC, Wang CJ. Mulberry leaf extract inhibits the development of atherosclerosis in cholesterol-fed rabbits and in cultures aortic vascular smooth muscle cells. Journal of Agricultural and Food Chemistry. 2013;**61**:2780-2788

[14] Chan KC, Ho HH, Peng CH, Lan KP, Lin MC, Chen HM, et al. Polyphenol-rich extract from mulberry leaf inhibits vascular smooth muscle cell proliferation involving upregulation of p53 and inhibition of cyclin-dependent kinase. Journal of Agricultural and Food Chemistry. 2010;**58**:2536-2542

[15] Yang MY, Chan KC, Lee YJ, Chang XZ, Wu CH, Wang CJ. Mulberry leaf polyphenol extract induced apoptosis involving regulation of adenosine monophosphate-activated protein kinase/fatty acid synthase in a p53-negative hepatocellular carcinoma cell. Journal of Agricultural and Food Chemistry. 2012;**60**:6891-6898

[16] Thomas J, Raj Kumar R, Mandal AKA. Metabolite profiling and characterization of somaclonal variants

in tea (*Camellia spp.*) for identifying productive and quality accession. Phytochemistry. 2006;**67**(11):1136-1142

[17] Rodriguez-Delgado MA, Malovana S, Perez JP, Borges T, Garcia-Montelongo FJ. Separation of phenolic compounds by high performance chromatography with absorbance and flurimetric detection. Journal of Chromatography. 2001;**912**:249-257

[18] Friedewald WT, Levy RI, Fredrickson DS. Estimation of the concentration of low-density lipoprotein cholesterol in plasma, without use of the preparative ultracentrifuge. Clinical Chemistry. 1972;**18**(6):499-502

[19] Morita T, Oh-hashi A, Takei K, Ikai M, Kasaoka S, Kiriyama S. Cholesterol-lowering effects of soybean, potato and rice proteins depend on their low methionine contents in rats fed a cholesterol-free purified diet. Journal of Nutrition. 1997;**127**(3):470-477

[20] Bancroft JD, Stevens A. Theory and Practice of Histological Techniques. London, UK: Longman Group; 1982

[21] Charrez B, Qiao L, Hebbard L. The role of fructose in metabolism and cancer. Hormone Molecular Biology and Clinical Investigation. 2015;**22**(2):79-89

[22] Bocarsly ME, Powell ES, Avena NM, Hoebel BG. High-fructose corn syrup causes characteristics of obesity in rats: Increased body weight, body fat and triglyceride levels. Pharmacology, Biochemistry and Behaviour. 2010;**97**(1):101-106

[23] Kals J, Kampus P, Kals M, Zilmer K, Kullisaar T, Teesalu R, et al. Impact of oxidative stress on arterial elasticity in patients with atherosclerosis. American Journal of Hypertension. 2006;**19**:902-908

[24] Smith SC Jr, Jackson R, Pearson TA, Fuster V, Yusuf S, Faergeman O. Principles for national and regional guidelines on cardiovascular disease prevention: A scientific statement from the World Heart and Stroke Forum. Circulation. 2004;**109**:3112-3121

[25] Yang XL, Yang L, Zheng HY. Hypolipidemic and antioxidant effects of mulberry (*Morus alba* L.) fruit in hyperlipidaemia rats. Food and Chemical Toxicology. 2010;**48**:2374-2379

[26] Chang YC, Yang MY, Chen SC, Wang CJ. Mulberry leaf polyphenol extract improves obesity by inducing adipocyte apoptosis and inhibiting preadipocyte differentiation and hepatic lipogenesis. Journal of Functional Foods. 2016;**21**:249-262

[27] Andallu B, Vinay Kumar AV, Varadacharyulu NC. Lipid abnormalities in streptozotocin-diabetes: Amelioration by *Morus indica* L. Cv Suguna leaves. International Journal of Diabetes in Developing Countries. 2009;**29**(3):123-128

[28] Enkhmaa B, Shiwaku K, Katsube T, Kitajima K, Anurad E, Yamasaki M, et al. Mulberry (*Morus alba* L.) leaves and their major flavonol quercetin-3-(6-malonylglucoside) attenuate atherosclerotic lesion development in LDL receptor-deficient mice. Journal of Nutrition. 2005;**135**:729-734

[29] Yang Y, Zhang Z, Li S, Ye X, Li X, He K. Synergy effects of herb extracts: pharmacokinetics and pharmacodynamic basis. Fitoterapia. 2014;**92**:133-147

[30] Wu CH, Lin MC, Wang HC, Yang MY, Jou MJ, Wang CJ. Rutin inhibits oleic acid induced lipid accumulation via reducing lipogenesis and oxidative stress in hepatocarcinoma cells. Journal of Food Science. 2011;**76**(2):T65-T72

[31] Sikder K, Kesh SB, Das N, Manna K, Dey S. The high antioxidative power

of quercetin (aglycone flavonoid) and its glycone (rutin) avert high cholesterol diet induced hepatotoxicity and inflammation in Swiss albino mice. Food and Function. 2014;**5**:1294-1303

[32] Sun X, Yamasaki M, Katsube T, Shiwaku K. Effects of quercetin derivatives from mulberry leaves: Improved gene expression related hepatic lipid and glucose metabolism in short-term high-fat fed mice. Nutrition Research and Practice. 2015;**9**:137-143

[33] Moon J, Do HJ, Kim OY, Shin MJ. Antiobesity effects of quercetin-rich onion peel extract on the differentiation of 3T3-L1 preadipocytes and the adipogenesis in high fat-fed rats. Food and Chemical Toxicology: An International Journal published for the British Industrial Biological Research Association. 2013;**58**:347-354

[34] Taher MA, Abdul-Hussain DA, Hasan HF, Fahmi ZM, Luaibi OK, Ali MG. Hypolipidemic effect of caffeic acid isolated from *Arctium lappa* cultivated in Iraq, in hyperlipidemic rat model. Iraqi Journal of Pharmaceutical Sciences. 2015;**24**(1):18-24

[35] Cho AS, Jeon SM, Kim MJ, Yeo J, Seo KI, Choi MS, et al. Chlorogenic acid exhibits anti-obesity property and improves lipid metabolism in high-fat diet-induced-obese mice. Food and Chemical Toxicology: An International Journal Published for the British Industrial Biological Research Association. 2010;**48**:937-943

[36] Yang MY, Chan KC, Lee YT, Chang XZ, Wu CH, Wang CJ. *Sechium edule* shoot extracts and active components improve obesity and a fatty liver that involved reducing hepatic lipogenesis and adipogenesis in high-fat diet-fed rats. Journal of Agricultural and Food Chemistry. 2015;**63**(18):4587-4596

[37] Liao CC, Ou TT, Huang HP, Wang CJ. The inhibition of oleic acid induced hepatic lipogenesis and the promotion of lipolysis by caffeic acid via up-regulation of AMP-activated kinase. Journal of the Science of Food and Agriculture. 2014;**94**:1154-1162

[38] Amalan V, Vijayakumar N, Indumathi D, Ramakrishnan A. Antidiabetic and antihyperlipidemic activity of p-coumaric acid in diabetic rats, role of pancreatic GLUT 2: *In vivo* approach. Biomedicine and Pharmacotherapy. 2016;**84**:230-236

[39] Tuovinen CG, Bender AE. Some metabolic effects of prolonged feeding of starch, sucrose, fructose and carbohydrate-free diet in the rat. Annals of Nutrition and Metabolism. 1975;**19**(3-4):161-172

[40] Marchesini G, Brizi M, Bianchi G, Tomassetti S, Bugianesi R, Lenzi M, et al. Nonalcoholic fatty liver disease—A feature of the metabolic syndrome. Diabetes. 2001;**50**:1844-1850

[41] Meli R, Raso GM, Irace C, Simeoli R, Di Pascale A, Paciello O, et al. High-fat diet induces liver steatosis and early dysregulation of iron metabolism in rats. PLoS One. 2013;**8**:e66570

[42] Chien MY, Ku YH, Chang JM, Yang CM, Chen CH. Effects of herbal mixture extracts on obesity in rats fed a high-fat diet. Journal of Food and Drug Analysis. 2016;**24**(3):594-601

Section 3

Nonalcoholic Fatty Liver Disease and Its Associated Parameters

Chapter 3

Insulin Therapy and Autoimmune Disease with Relevance to Non Alchoholic Fatty Liver Disease

Ian James Martins

Abstract

The diabetes epidemic is now expected by the year 2050 to become a global pandemic with approx. 592 million affected in both the developed and developing world. The treatment of diabetes by insulin therapy has been the focus for many diabetics with the improvement and prevention of various diseases such as cardiovascular disease, kidney disease and neurodegeneration. The global nonalcoholic fatty liver disease (NAFLD) epidemic has now become of major concern to diabetes with critical interest in insulin therapy to reverse and stabilize autoimmune disease with relevance to NAFLD and the diabetes pandemic. Dietary components that activate anti-aging genes improve insulin therapy and should be assessed with specific amounts and doses of Indian spices consumed that may not interfere with insulin therapy and induce mitophagy in various diseases. Food quality, appetite control and core body temperature are critical to maintain insulin therapy with unhealthy diets linked to NAFLD and diabetes. Genomic medicine and dietary activators are essential to maintain insulin therapy and prevent toxic immune reactions with relevance to NAFLD and diabetes management.

Keywords: insulin therapy, genomic, autoimmune disease, diabetes, global, mitophagy, curcumin, cinnamon

1. Introduction

The diabetes epidemic is expected to affect approx. 592 people by the year 2035. The urgency to prevent the largest diabetes epidemic in history has now assessed multiple risk factors involved with induction of Type 3 diabetes connected to various chronic diseases. Insulin resistance and brain aging now indicate neuron vulnerability to mitophagy associated with the diabetes pandemic expected in 2050 [1, 2]. Diabetes and its connections autoimmunity [3] have become important to mitophagy, metabolic disease with relevance to the nonalcoholic fatty liver disease (NAFLD) epidemic.

An association between various genes and the immune system [4, 5] has been proposed to be involved with the regulation of life-span in various species. Immune gene activation has been associated with brain aging [6] with the critical involvement of inflammation in the development of neuro-degeneration. Autoimmune disease, drugs and immunosenescence are related to the chronic disease epidemic with uncontrolled release of inflammatory cytokines such as tumor necrosis factor

IntechOpen

α and interleukin-6 [7, 8]. Major interests to determine human longevity require the assessment of nutrition and diet with relevance to the control of inflammatory cytokines that are associated with age-related changes in the immune system and the induction of diabetes, NAFLD and neurodegeneration.

Appetite control with relevance to immuno-metabolism has become critical to the treatment of NAFLD. The major defect in global chronic disease is autoimmune disease with defective adipose tissue and liver interaction involved with the release of inflammatory cytokines and adipo-cytokines relevant to toxic immune reactions that involve the pancreas, brain, heart, thyroid, kidneys and reproductive organs. Appetite control and autoimmune disease are connected to anti-aging genes with relevance to irreversible programmed cell death in various cells and tissues. Immune competence changes over a human's life span with a process known as immunosenescence [9, 10]. In man multiple theories of aging have been proposed with the immune theory of aging that involve abnormal inflammatory responses that contribute to the induction of chronic diseases [11].

In various communities in the developing and developed world the understanding of the ingestion of a healthy diet and hepatic fat metabolism has become of critical importance to the treatment diabetes that is now linked to various organ diseases. In the world [12] transition to healthy diets has become urgent to prevent insulin resistance, autoimmune disease and NAFLD. The liver is the major organ for the metabolism of dietary fat and after consumption of a meal in healthy individuals the fat is rapidly metabolized by the mitochondria in the liver.

A diet rich in fat and sugar that lead to fat deposition in the liver can be referred to as liver steatosis. The defect in the liver fatty acid metabolism is possibly related to mitochondrial dysfunction and a careful calorie controlled diet may reverse liver steatosis. As mitochondrial apoptosis occurs steatohepatitis may be associated with liver inflammation. Steatohepatitis may induce NAFLD that may then progress to severe inflammation and liver cirrhosis. In obesity and diabetes the metabolism of a fat meal by the liver is defective with associated hyperglycemia and hyperinsulinemia. Food restriction [13] and appetite control are vital to the treatment of NAFLD with hepatic fat metabolism connected to insulin resistance, autoimmune disease and mitophagy [14].

2. Diabetes and pathogenetic loop complications

Insulin treatment in diabetes has provided information that approx. 30% of patients are involved with insulin treatment or plan to start insulin with insulin regimens [15] associated with various insulin doses and failure of oral anti-diabetic medications. Type 2 diabetes mellitus is characterized by hyperglycemia, insulin resistance, and impairment of insulin secretion [16]. The impairment of insulin secretion is related to hyperglycemia, high serum low-density lipoprotein cholesterol concentrations and low serum high-density lipoprotein cholesterol concentrations with relevance to cardiovascular disease [17]. The relative importance of impaired insulin release and insulin resistance in the pathogenesis of Type 2 diabetes has been evaluated and may be connected to NAFLD. NAFLD may be connected to autoimmune disease and mitophagy associated with impairment in insulin secretion and cardiovascular disease [18–20]. In Type 1 diabetes the use of insulin therapy has been assessed with the critical importance to reduce hyperglycemia, severe hypoglycemia and the development of long-term complications [21–23]. Insulin therapy should be carefully evaluated in Type 1 and Type 2 diabetes with relevance to reduction in plasma glucose levels [24]. Interference in hepatic glucose production [24, 25] or interference with increased glucose uptake by the liver may be sensitive to repression

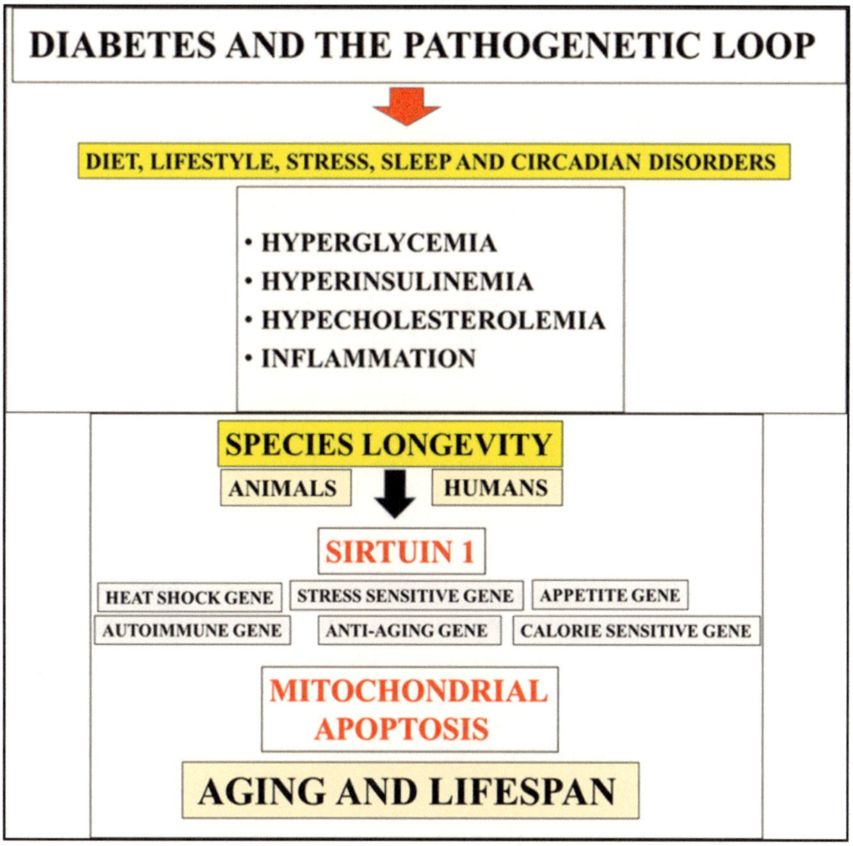

Figure 1.
Diabetes and the pathogenetic loop associated with inflammation, age related diseases and neurodegeneration involve inactivation of the anti-aging gene Sirtuin 1 (Sirt 1) associated with mitochondrial apoptosis in various species and man.

of glucose related genes associated with the induction of glucolipotoxicity, NAFLD and insulin resistance. Exercise and insulin therapy [26] may reduce glucolipotoxicity and NAFLD but with the aging process the pathogenetic loop [27–32] that involve hyperglycemia, hypercholesterolemia and hyperinsulinemia may be associated with autoimmune disease, mitophagy and programmed cell death of various cells and tissues [18–20]. The role of diet, lifestyle, stress, sleep and circadian disorders [33] may inactivate the anti-aging gene Sirtuin 1 (Sirt 1) with relevance to insulin therapy and induction of NAFLD associated with the pathogenetic loop (**Figure 1**) and uncontrolled inflammation of cells and tissues [18–20].

3. Anti-aging genes, mitochondrial apoptosis and programmed cell death

Insulin resistance is involved early in alterations of nuclear, subcellular and cell membrane function that lead to cell transformation without reversible changes with accelerated cell apoptosis [34]. In 2050 the predicted global diabetes pandemic [1, 2] has accelerated scientific research to determine the identification of novel genomic pathways such as the anti-aging gene Sirt 1 that may provide new knowledge with relevance to accelerated cell apoptosis and inactivated insulin therapy. In Type 2 diabetes and Type 1 diabetes various genes and genetic loci have been reported to be involved in the development of diabetes [35]. Novel genes [36] have been identified that are involved with autoimmune disease [18, 19, 36, 37] and glucolipotoxicity with irreversible immune complications relevant to NAFLD, diabetes [3] and the pathogenetic loop. The discovery of the anti-aging gene Sirt 1 now has become important to the treatment of diabetes with insulin therapy in Type 1 and Type 2 diabetes connected to Sirt 1 activation in the pancreas with relevance to insulin release [38] with Sirt 1 associated with mitochondrial biogenesis (**Figure 1**) and cell survival in various tissues [38, 39]. The inactivation of Sirt 1 [39] in humans leads to the pathogenetic loop in diabetes and implicates nutritional and environmental factors in the induction of programmed cell death.

Sirt 1 is a nicotinamide adenine dinucleotide (NAD+) dependent class III histone deacetylase (HDAC) that targets transcription factors such as p 53 to adapt gene expression to metabolic activity and the deacetylation of nuclear receptors indicate its critical involvement in insulin resistance and autoimmune disease [18]. In situ hybridization analysis has localized the human Sirt 1 gene to chromosome 10q21.3 [18]. Calorie restriction is essential for Sirt 1 transcriptional regulation with other factors such as diet and lifestyle critical for the prevention of insulin resistance and NAFLD. Sirt 1 is an acute phase protein involved with neuron proliferation [18] and its regulation of the suprachiasmatic nucleus is involved with control of the circadian rhythm [18]. The circadian rhythm and immune system are closely connected to the immune response. Nutritional interventions that are controlled by the consumption of a low calorie diet indicate the maintenance of connections between Sirt 1 and other anti-aging genes such as Klotho, p66shc (longevity protein) and FOXO1/FOXO3a that are connected to programmed cell death [36]. Sirt 1 and transcriptional regulation of anti-aging genes are critical to mitophagy (**Figure 1**) and neurodegenerative disease with accelerated brain aging connected to NAFLD and diabetes [19, 36].

4. Insulin therapy and Indian spices with relevance to NAFLD and diabetes

The connections between NAFLD and diabetes have become of central importance to the expected diabetes pandemic by the year 2050 [1, 2]. NAFLD in diabetic individuals may completely inactivate insulin therapy with defective insulin dose regimens and failure of oral anti-diabetic medications. The defect in the liver fatty acid metabolism is possibly related to mitochondrial dysfunction associated with severe liver inflammation and steatohepatitis that may induce NAFLD that may then progress to severe inflammation (NASH) and liver cirrhosis. Insulin therapy has been used to improve liver function but with NAFLD, high dose insulin therapy may be unsuccessful with liver inflammation [40–42] associated with uncontrolled hyperglycemia and mitochondrial apoptosis (**Figure 2**). Insulin therapy with insulin dose and oral anti-diabetic medications should be re-evaluated to improve hepatocyte mitochondrial biogenesis with relevance to reversal of liver disease connected to hyperglycemia and NAFLD in various Type 1, Type 2 and Type 3 [35, 39] diabetics.

The connections between Sirt 1 and insulin resistance have accelerated in recent years with Sirt 1 as a calorie sensitive gene is now implicated in insulin resistance and to the important to glucose dependent insulin secretion with protection of pancreatic β-cell mass [43–46]. Sirt 1 may be involved in silencing insulin resistance by regulation of specific proteins involved in insulin action [47]. Anti-inflammatory actions in adipocytes involve Sirt 1 repression and inflammation [48, 49] associated with the adipose-liver defect [49, 50] and the induction of NAFLD. Sirt 1

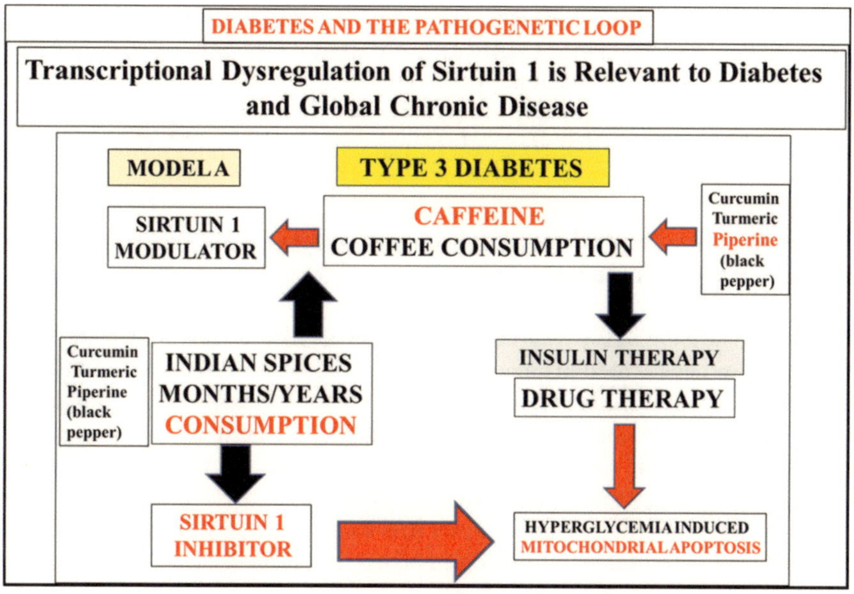

Figure 2.
Indian spices have become important as a diabetes technology and its use in diabetes has become of concern. Indian spices such as curcumin and cinnamon associated with glucose control in diabetics but excessive curcumin or piperine may inactivate insulin therapy associated with hyperglycemic induced mitochondrial apoptosis in the brain and the periphery.

dysfunction in the brain leads to systemic insulin resistance [51] with close links to Type 3 diabetes and NAFLD [52, 53]. In Sirt 1 knockout mice increased adipose tissue mass has been connected to NAFLD [33]. The expression of Sirt 1 protein has a molecular weight (Mol Wt) of 81 kda with Mol Wt variation (81–110 kda). Insulin therapy to prevent NAFLD requires insulin dose/antidiabetic medication calculation to release the Sirt 1 acute phase protein [18, 37]. Sirt 1 is essential to prevent inflammation and Sirt 1 inactivation may induce NAFLD that may corrupt pancreas function. Insulin therapy and plasma Sirt 1 levels may allow mitochondrial biogenesis to be assessed with relevance to therapeutic glucose control in Type 1, 2 and 3 diabetics. It is unclear if inactivation of insulin therapy is associated with mitophagy and the induction of NAFLD and various organ diseases [52]. Appetite control [13, 18] is now critical to the maintenance of mitochondrial biogenesis and insulin therapy with overeating [13] connected to inactivation of insulin therapy and linked to the severity of the diabetic condition.

Indian spices have become important as a diabetes technology [54] with Indian spices such as curcumin and cinnamon associated with glucose control in diabetics (**Figure 2**). The event of insulin therapy as the primary therapy in diabetes technology has raised concern with relevance to the consumption of Indian spices as a secondary technology [55]. Indian spices consumed over many years are not cleared from the body and may bind to cells and receptors with excess Indian spices that may associate with insulin receptors related to altered insulin actions and inactivated insulin therapy. In normal individuals consumption of cinnamon and curcumin may inactivate the biological activity of insulin [54, 55] with Indian spices as the secondary treatment for glucose control in the brain and the periphery. Drugs such as anti-obese drugs [56] and novel drugs [57] are now of critical importance to NAFLD and insulin therapy. Insulin therapy and the use of various therapeutic drugs in diabetes have been linked to the treatment of organ dysfunction [35, 57–59] in diabetes. The use of Indian spices should be reassessed in various populations to prevent interference with drug/insulin therapy (**Figure 2**) or with caffeine effects [60] relevant to the treatment of NAFLD and diabetes. The mixing of spices such as curcumin, turmeric and black pepper in coffee should be discouraged and may contribute to the transcriptional dysregulation of Sirt 1 and induction of mitochondrial apoptosis relevant to diabetes and the pathogenetic loop [27–32].

5. Genomic medicine and Sirt 1 activators reverse immune reactions in global chronic disease

Genomic medicine in the treatment of cardiovascular disease and diabetes [19, 37] has now accelerated in various communities. Peripheral nutrition is essential early to prevent neurodegeneration (Type 3 diabetes) that lead to uncontrolled peripheral glucose homeostasis. Type 3 diabetes is associated with suprachiasmatic nucleus defects with the abnormal maintenance of brain and whole body glucose metabolism in various species and man [20]. Nutritional therapy in diabetics now need to involve the use of Sirt 1 activators [61] to prevent the effects of various Sirt 1 inhibitors that accumulate in the blood plasma that repress Sirt 1 expression in cells and tissues. A dose of 4 g/day of phosphatidylinositol [62] is essential with insulin therapy to prevent hyperglycemia, NAFLD and other neurodegenerative diseases. Sirt 1 inhibitors such as excess palmitic acid (cream, cheese), alcohol and drugs (suramin and sirtinol) should be carefully controlled to prevent inactivation of insulin therapy. Sirt 1 activators such as pyruvic acid, leucine and magnesium are critical with relevance to insulin therapy. Diabetic individuals with Indian spice consumption (**Figure 3**) over years need to be carefully evaluated with relevance to plasma Sirt 1 inhibitors, xenobiotics [63], caffeine content [60], drug therapy, bacterial lipopolysaccharides (LPS) and mycotoxins [62] that may interfere with insulin/oral medication therapy. The importance of genomic medicine may indicate that the immune system may malfunction [37] early with relevance to poor nutrition of food quality with irreversible organ disease manifestations. Biotherapy and the immune system [37, 61] may be critical to insulin therapy and connected to insulin resistance and NAFLD. Appetite control and essential food components [64] may be essential to maintain the immune system with autoimmune disease

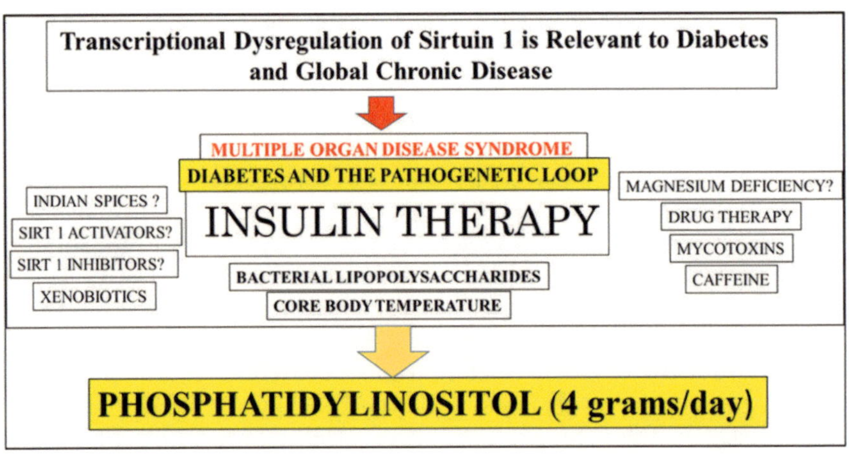

Figure 3.
Poor food quality and core body temperature defects will inactivate Sirt 1 and induce insulin resistance and NAFLD. Sirt 1 inhibitors such as xenobiotics, caffeine/Indian spice over-consumption and magnesium deficiency may lead to the diabetes pandemic with high doses of phosphatidylinositol essential to maintain insulin therapy and prevent the induction of NAFLD.

associated with appetite dysregulation and poor food quality. Specific mitochondrial nutrients [65] with insulin therapy need to be consumed to prevent severe mitophagy and organ disease.

Food quality with relevance to stroke, synaptic plasticity and neurological diseases has become important to diabetic individuals with essential maintenance and prevention of brain diseases by insulin therapy. Unhealthy diets that contain LPS, mycotoxins and xenobiotics can induce NAFLD with inactivation of insulin therapy. In the developing world increased plasma LPS levels (**Figure 3**) have raised concern with relevance to induction of metabolic and neurodegenerative diseases [66, 67]. Antibiotic resistance with relevance to antimicrobial drug use should be carefully controlled to prevent excessive release of LPS from the debris of gram negative bacteria [68]. Food preparation should be carefully assessed to prevent end products such as LPS and patulin that may persist in contaminated food [63, 69]. LPS and patulin may inactivate Sirt 1 [62] with relevance to insulin resistance and NAFLD. Xenobiotics [63] in air, food and water may inactivate insulin therapy (**Figure 3**) with increased xenobiotic levels associated with mitochondrial apoptosis.

Core body temperature (**Figure 3**) and insulin therapy are closely connected and dysregulation of core body temperature may induce NAFLD. The discovery of the heat shock gene Sirt 1 [70] has indicated that careful body temperature control is critical to prevent autoimmune disease and mitochondrial apoptosis. Sirt 1 and its inactivation are associated with increased heat shock protein 70 with relevance to natural killer cell activation and mitochondrial apoptosis. Nutritional therapy and core body temperature are essential to maintain insulin therapy in diabetics with relevance to mitophagy and programmed cell death. The event of heat shock protein 70 disturbances may lead to kidney injury [71] and associated with chronic kidney disease and neurodegeneration in diabetes.

6. Novel biomarkers and insulin therapy may reverse NAFLD and diabetes

The analysis of various plasma biomarkers with insulin therapy [72] has become of major interest to NAFLD development, therapeutic strategies [73–77] and diabetes research. Essential measurements of plasma Sirt 1 and heat shock protein levels need to be determined to indicate core body temperature defects with relevance to inactivation of insulin therapy. Tissue analysis of anti-aging genes [18, 33, 54] need to be conducted to determine the role of insulin therapy with relevance to reversal of NAFLD [18, 33, 35, 49, 55, 68, 69] with connections to inflammation and metabolic diseases. Plasma assays of inflammatory cytokines such as tumor necrosis factor alpha, interleukin-1 and interleukin-6 [10, 11] need to be assayed with effective insulin therapy. The major limitation with insulin therapy is to correlate the dose of insulin injected with plasma biomarkers [78] that maintain mitochondrial biogenesis associated with the prevention of NAFLD (**Figure 4**). The use of antimicrobials [79] with insulin therapy should be carefully controlled to prevent increased release of gram negative bacteria LPS end products that may interfere with glucose homeostasis and induce NAFLD. Plasma LPS should be measured with antimicrobial use in individuals on insulin therapy. The connections between the antimicrobial activity, immune system and nitric oxide homeostasis involve Sirt 1 and connected to toxic immune reactions [80].

The geriatric population in many communities is associated with insulin resistance, Sirt 1 repression and nuclear-mitochondria defects relevant to NAFLD. Sirt 1 measurement in the plasma, cytoplasm and nucleus are essential to determine

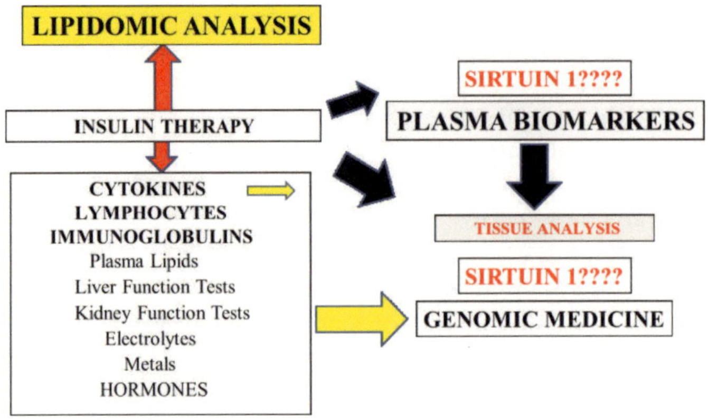

Figure 4.
Complications of insulin therapy in diabetes lead to irreversible mitophagy and programmed cell death with relevance to defective Sirt 1 expression in diabetic individuals. Conventional clinical biochemistry tests do not indicate nuclear-mitochondria defects associated with autoimmune disease and mitophagy but lipidomic tests may be relevant to insulin therapy and Sirt 1 analysis.

the relevance of insulin therapy and mitochondrial apoptosis when compared to the validity of various diagnostic tests and plasma analytic measurements. In many biomarker laboratories the comprehensive assessment of various biomarkers may not be correlated with insulin therapy with mitophagy the inevitable cellular defect in geriatric individuals. Analysis of plasma biomarkers (**Figure 4**) and tissue samples may indicate a primary autoimmune reaction related to a defective nuclear-mitochondria interaction.

Insulin therapy and its use should be carefully revised with relevance to conventional plasma tests that do not indicate cellular mitophagy and toxic immune reactions associated with diabetes [81, 82]. Previous studies [83, 84] with the assessment of the role of insulin on cytokines, lymphocytes and macrophages do not assess Sirt 1's role in toxic immune reactions and mitophagy. Recent studies have shown that molecular lipid biomarkers from lipidomic analysis [85–88] may determine diabetes severity. The role of insulin therapy with relevance to lipidomic biomarkers may integrate routine plasma biomarker testing with relevance to cellular Sirt 1 expression and plasma Sirt 1 analysis (**Figure 4**).

7. Conclusion

Insulin treatment has been evaluated in diabetes but the global NAFLD epidemic that is expected to reach between 20 and 30% of the worldwide communities will now be connected to diabetes pandemic and the pathogenetic loop. Insulin therapy has been assessed with relevance to improvement in inflammatory conditions but the defect in the anti-aging gene Sirt 1 and diabetic mitophagy still persists with the induction of NAFLD and various organ diseases. Insulin therapy with Indian spice consumption requires reassessment to avoid over-consumption of Indian spices that may inactivate insulin therapy and mitochondrial biogenesis. Food quality, appetite control and core body temperature are critical to maintain insulin therapy with unhealthy diets linked to NAFLD and diabetes. Genomic medicine and Sirt 1 activators are essential to maintain insulin therapy in the developing world with toxic immune reactions important to NAFLD. Insulin therapy may not reverse the nuclear-mitochondria defect that is relevant to global organ disease and various plasma biomarkers.

Acknowledgements

This work was supported by grants from Edith Cowan University, the McCusker Alzheimer's Research Foundation and the National Health and Medical Research Council.

Abbreviations

NAFLD	nonalcoholic fatty liver disease
Sirt 1	Sirtuin 1
LPS	bacterial lipopolysaccharides

Author details

Ian James Martins[1,2,3]*

1 Centre of Excellence in Alzheimer's Disease Research and Care, Sarich Neuroscience Research Institute, Edith Cowan University, Nedlands, Western Australia, Australia

2 School of Psychiatry and Clinical Neurosciences, The University of Western Australia, Nedlands, Australia

3 McCusker Alzheimer's Research Foundation, Hollywood Medical Centre, Nedlands, Australia

*Address all correspondence to: i.martins@ecu.edu.au

IntechOpen

© 2018 The Author(s). Licensee IntechOpen. This chapter is distributed under the terms of the Creative Commons Attribution License (http://creativecommons.org/licenses/by/3.0), which permits unrestricted use, distribution, and reproduction in any medium, provided the original work is properly cited.

References

[1] Zimmet PZ. Diabetes and its drivers: The largest epidemic in human history? Clinical Diabetes and Endocrinology. 2017;**3**:1

[2] Zimmet PZ, Alberti KG. Epidemiology of diabetes-status of a pandemic and issues around metabolic surgery. Diabetes Care. 2016;**39**:878-883

[3] Michels AW, Eisenbarth GS. Immunologic endocrine disorders. Journal of Allergy and Clinical Immunology. 2010;**125**:S226-S237

[4] Gruver AL, Hudson LL, Sempowski GD. Immunosenescence of ageing. The Journal of Pathology. 2007;**211**:144-156

[5] Vasto S, Caruso C. Immunity and ageing: A new journal looking at ageing from an immunological point of view. Immunity and Ageing. 2004;**1**:1

[6] Fulop T, Witkowski JM, Pawelec G, Alan C, Larbi A. On the immunological theory of aging. Interdisciplinary Topics in Gerontology. 2014;**39**:163-176

[7] Passarino G, De Rango F, Montesanto A. Human longevity: Genetics or lifestyle? It takes two to tango. Immunity and Ageing. 2016;**13**:12

[8] Doria G, Frasca D. Genetic factors in immunity and aging. Vaccine. 2000;**18**:1591-1595

[9] Cribbs DH, Berchtold NC, Perreau V, Coleman PD, Rogers J, Tenner AJ, et al. Extensive innate immune gene activation accompanies brain aging, increasing vulnerability to cognitive decline and neurodegeneration: A microarray study. Journal of Neuroinflammation. 2012;**9**:179

[10] Kulmatycki KM, Jamali F. Drug disease interactions: Role of inflammatory mediators in disease and variability in drug response. Journal of Pharmacy and Pharmaceutical Sciences. 2005;**8**:602-625

[11] Lai Y, Dong C. Therapeutic antibodies that target inflammatory cytokines in autoimmune diseases. International Immunology. 2016;**28**:181-188

[12] Alam S, Mustafa G, Alam M, Ahmad N. Insulin resistance in development and progression of nonalcoholic fatty liver disease. World Journal of Gastrointestinal Pathophysiology. 2016;**7**:211-217

[13] Martins IJ. In: Jones E, editor. Appetite Dysregulation and Obesity in Western Countries. Saarbrucken, Deutschland/Germany: LAP LAMBERT Academic Publishing; 2013. ISBN: 978-3-659-40372-9

[14] Martins IJ. Autoimmune disease and mitochondrial dysfunction in chronic diseases. Research Chronic Diseases. 2017;**1**:10-12

[15] Davidson MB. Insulin therapy: A personal approach. Clinical Diabetes. 2015;**33**:123-135

[16] Kramer CK, Zinman B, Retnakaran R. Short-term intensive insulin therapy in type 2 diabetes mellitus: A systematic review and meta-analysis. Lancet Diabetes and Endocrinology. 2013;**1**:28-34

[17] Silver B, Ramaiya K, Andrew SB, Fredrick O, Bajaj S, Kalra S, et al. EADSG guidelines: Insulin therapy in diabetes. Diabetes Therapeutics. 2018;**9**:449-492

[18] Martins IJ. Appetite control and biotherapy in the Management of Autoimmune Induced Global Chronic Diseases. Journal of Clinical Immunology and Research. 2018;**2**:1-4

[19] Martins IJ. Genomic medicine and acute cardiovascular disease progression

in diabetes. International Journal of Medical Studies. 2018;**3**:124-130

[20] Martins IJ. Insulin therapy inactivation is connected to NAFLD and diabetes severity index. Journal of Diabetes and Clinical Studies. 2017;**1**:001-003

[21] Campbell MD, Walker M, Bracken RM, Turner D, Stevenson RJ, Gonzalez JT, et al. Insulin therapy and dietary adjustments to normalize glycemia and prevent nocturnal hypoglycemia after evening exercise in type 1 diabetes: A randomized controlled trial. BMJ Open Diabetes Research and Care. 2015;**3**:e000085

[22] Yadav S, Parakh A. Insulin therapy. Indian Pediatrics. 2006;**43**:863-872

[23] Lechleitner M, Hoppichler F. Insulin therapy. Wiener Medizinische Wochenschrift. 2011;**161**:300-304

[24] DeWitt DE, Hirsch IB. Outpatient insulin therapy in type 1 and type 2 diabetes mellitus: Scientific review. The Journal of the American Medical Association. 2003;**289**:2254-2264

[25] Mudaliar S, Edelman SV. Insulin therapy in type 2 diabetes. Endocrinology and Metabolism Clinics of North America. 2001;**30**:935-982

[26] Kourtoglou GI. Insulin therapy and exercise. Diabetes Research and Clinical Practice. 2011;**93**:S73-S77

[27] Kohei K. Pathophysiology of type 2 diabetes and its treatment policy research and reviews. Journal of the Japan Medical Association. 2010;**53**:41-46

[28] Leahy JL. Pathogenesis of type 2 diabetes mellitus. Archives of Medical Research. 2005;**36**:197-209

[29] Cersosimo E, Triplitt C, Solis-Herrera C, et al. Pathogenesis of type 2 diabetes mellitus. In: De Groot LJ, Chrousos G, Dungan K, et al., editors. Endotext [Internet]. South Dartmouth, MA: MDText.com, Inc.; 2000 Available from: https://www.ncbi.nlm.nih.gov/books/NBK279115/

[30] McCulloch DK. Pathogenesis of type 2 diabetes mellitus—UpToDate. 2016. Available from: https://www.uptodate.com/contents/pathogenesis-of-type-2-diabetes-mellitus

[31] DeFronzo RA, Ferrannini E, Zimmet P, George K, Alberti MM. Pathogenesis of type 2 diabetes mellitus. In: Chapter 25 Published Print: 17 April 2015 International Textbook of Diabetes Mellitus. 4th ed. United Kingdom: John Wiley & Sons, Ltd; ISBN: 9781118387658

[32] Kahn SE, Cooper ME, Del Prato S. Pathophysiology and treatment of type 2 diabetes: Perspectives on the past, present, and future. Lancet. 2014;**383**:1068-1083

[33] Martins IJ. Induction of NAFLD with increased risk of obesity and chronic diseases in developed countries. Open Journal of Endocrine and Metabolic Diseases. 2014; **4**:90-110

[34] Martins IJ. Diabetes and organ dysfunction in the developing and developed. World Global Journal of Medical Research: F Diseases. 2015;**15**:15-21

[35] Martins IJ. Diet and nutrition reverse type 3 diabetes and accelerated aging linked to global chronic diseases. Journal of Diabetes Research and Therapy. 2016;**2**:1-6

[36] Martins IJ. Anti-aging genes improve appetite regulation and reverse cell senescence and apoptosis in global populations. Advances in Aging Research. 2016;**5**:9-26

[37] Martins IJ. Genomic medicine and endocrine autoimmunity as key to mitochondrial disease. Global Journal of Endocrinological Metabolism. 2018;**2**:1-3

[38] Bordone L, Motta MC, Picard F, Robinson A, Jhala US, Apfeld J, et al. Sirt1 regulates insulin secretion by repressing UCP2 in pancreatic β cells. PLoS Biology. 2006;**4**:e31

[39] Martins IJ. Anti-aging gene linked to appetite regulation determines longevity in humans and animals. International Journal of Aging Research. 2018;**1**:1-4

[40] Jeschke MG, Klein D, Herndon DH. Insulin treatment improves the systemic inflammatory reaction to severe trauma. Annal of Surgery. 2004;**239**:553-560

[41] Chen Z, Yu R, Xiong Y, Du F, Zhu S. A vicious circle between insulin resistance and inflammation in nonalcoholic fatty liver disease. Lipids in Health and Disease. 2017;**16**:203

[42] Dal S, Jeandidier N, Seyfritz E, Bietiger W, Péronet C, Moreau F, et al. Featured article: Oxidative stress status and liver tissue defenses in diabetic rats during intensive subcutaneous insulin therapy. Experimental Biology and Medicine (Maywood). 2016;**241**:184-192

[43] Cao Y, Jiang X, Ma H, Wang Y, Xue P, Liu Y. SIRT1 and insulin resistance. The Journal of Diabetic Complications. 2016;**30**:178-183

[44] Liang F, Kume S, Koya D. SIRT1 and insulin resistance. Nature Reveiws in Endocrinology. 2009;**5**:367-373

[45] Yoshizaki T, Milne JC, Imamura T, Schenk S, Sonoda N, Babendure JL, et al. SIRT1 exerts anti-inflammatory effects and improves insulin sensitivity in adipocytes. Molecular and Cellular Biology. 2009;**29**:1363-1374

[46] Zabolotny JM, Kim YB. Silencing insulin resistance through SIRT1. Cell Metabolism. 2007;**6**:247-249

[47] de Luca C, Olefsky JM. Inflammation and insulin resistance. FEBS Letters. 2008;**582**:97-105

[48] Wieser V, Moschen AR, Tilg H. Inflammation, cytokines and insulin resistance: A clinical perspective. Archivum Immunologiae et Therapia Experimentalis (Warsz). 2013;**61**:119-125

[49] Martins IJ. Unhealthy Nutrigenomic diets accelerate NAFLD and adiposity in global communities. Journal of Molecular and Genetic Medicine. 2015;**9**:1

[50] Martins IJ. Defective interplay between adipose tissue and immune system induces non alcoholic fatty liver disease. Updates in Nutritional Disorders and Therapy. 2017;**1**:1-6

[51] Lu M, Sarruf DA, Li P, Osborn O, Sanchez-Alavez M, Talukdar S, et al. Neuronal Sirt1 deficiency increases insulin sensitivity in both brain and peripheral tissues. Journal of Biological Chemistry. 2013;**288**:10722-10735

[52] Martins IJ. Type 3 diabetes with links to NAFLD and other chronic diseases in the Western world. International Journal of Diabetes. 2016;**1**:1-5

[53] Martins IJ. Heat shock gene Sirtuin 1 regulates post-prandial lipid metabolism with relevance to nutrition and appetite regulation in diabetes. International Journal of Diabetes and Clinical Diagnosis. International Journal of Diabetes and Clinical Diagnosis. 2016;**3**:20

[54] Martins IJ. Indian spices and insulin therapy in diabetes and neurodegenerative diseases. Journal of Diabetes and Clinical Studies. 2018;**1**:1-3

[55] Martins IJ. Indian spices and biotherapeutics in health and chronic disease. Health. 2018;**10**:374-380

[56] Martins IJ. Drug therapy for obesity with anti-aging genes modification. Annals of Obesity and Disorders. 2016;**1**:1001

[57] Cole BK, Feaver RE, Wamhoff BR, Dash A. Non-alcoholic fatty liver disease (NAFLD) models in drug discovery. Expert Opinion in Drug Discovery. 2018;**13**:193-205

[58] Martins IJ. Sirtuin 1, a diagnostic protein marker and its relevance to chronic disease and therapeutic drug interventions. EC Pharmacology and Toxicology. 2018;**6.4**:209-215

[59] Martins IJ. Indian spices and unhealthy diets interfere with drug therapy in diabetes and neurodegenerative diseases. Novel Approaches in Drug Designing and Development. 2018;**3**:555616

[60] Martins IJ. Indian spices and caffeine treatment for obesity and cardiovascular disease. Annals of Clinical Endocrinology and Metabolism. 2018;**2**:010-014

[61] Martins IJ. Biotherapy and the immune system in ageing science. Acta Scientific Nutritional Health. 2018;**2**(**4**):29-31

[62] Martins IJ. Overnutrition determines LPS regulation of mycotoxin induced neurotoxicity in neurodegenerative diseases. International Journal of Molecular Sciences. 2015;**16**:29554-29573

[63] Martins IJ. Chapter 01. Increased risk for obesity and diabetes with neurodegeneration in developing countries. In: Top 10 Contribution on Genetics. Book Chapter. Avid Science.2018. www.avid.science.com

[64] Martins IJ. Functional foods and active molecules with relevance to health and chronic disease: Editorial. Functional Foods in Health and Disease. 2017;**7**:833-836

[65] Martins IJ. The global obesity epidemic is related to stroke, dementia and Alzheimer's disease. JSM Alzheimer's Disease and Related Dementia. 2014;**1**:1010

[66] Martins IJ. Bacterial lipopolysaccharides and neuron toxicity in neurodegenerative diseases. Neurology and Neurosurgery. 2018;**1**:1-3

[67] Martins IJ. Bacterial lipopolysaccharides change membrane fluidity with relevance to phospholipid and amyloid Beta dynamics in Alzheimer's disease. Journal of Microbial and Biochemical Technology. 2016;**8**:322-324

[68] Martins IJ. Antibiotic resistance involves antimicrobial inactivation in global communities. SAJ Pharmaacy and Pharmacology. 2017;**2**:102

[69] Martins IJ. Food quality induces a miscible disease with relevance to Alzheimer's disease and neurological diseases. Journal of Food Research. 2016;**5**:45-52

[70] Martins IJ. Heat shock gene inactivation and protein aggregation with links to chronic diseases. Diseases. 2018;**6**:1-5

[71] Martins IJ. Heat shock protein aggregation and chronic kidney disease. Research on Chronic Diseases. 2018;**2**:42-44

[72] Martins IJ. Advances in biomarkers and insulin therapy with relevance to reversal of diabetes. Journal of Studies on Diabetes. 2018;**1**:9-14

[73] Kitade H, Chen G, Ni Y, Ota T. Nonalcoholic fatty liver disease and

insulin resistance: New insights and potential new treatments. Nutrients. 2017;**9**:pii: E387

[74] Mills EP, Brown KPD, Smith JD, Vang PW, Trotta K. Treating nonalcoholic fatty liver disease in patients with type 2 diabetes mellitus: A review of efficacy and safety. Therapeutic Advances in Endocrinology and Metabolism. 2018;**9**:15-28

[75] Issa D, Patel V, Sanyal AJ. Future therapy for non-alcoholic fatty liver disease. Liver International. 2018;**38**:56-63

[76] Friedman SL, Neuschwander-Tetri BA, Rinella M, Sanyal AJ. Mechanisms of NAFLD development and therapeutic strategies. Nature Medicine. 2018;**24**:908-922

[77] Sumida Y, Yoneda M. Current and future pharmacological therapies for NAFLD/NASH. Journal of Gastroenterology. 2018;**53**:362-376

[78] Lees T, Nassif N, Simpson A, Shad-Kaneez F, Martiniello-Wilks R, Lin Y, et al. Recent advances in molecular biomarkers for diabetes mellitus: A systematic review. Biomarkers. 2017;**22**:604-613

[79] Dos Reis SA, do Carmo Gouveia Peluzio M, Bressan J. The use of antimicrobials as adjuvant therapy for the treatment of obesity and insulin resistance: Effects and associated mechanisms. Diabetes/Metabolism Research and Reveiws. 2018 Apr 16:e3014. [Epub ahead of print]

[80] Martins IJ. Antimicrobial activity inactivation and toxic immune reactions induce epilepsy in human. Journal of Medical Discovery. 2017;**2**:jmd17040

[81] Itariu BK, Stulnig TM. Autoimmune aspects of type 2 diabetes mellitus—A mini-review. Gerontology. 2014;**60**: 189-196

[82] Hemminki K, Liu X, Försti A, Sundquist J, Sundquist K, Ji J. Subsequent type 2 diabetes in patients with autoimmune disease. Scientific Reports. 2015;**5**:13871

[83] Nell LJ, Thomas JW. The human immune response to insulin. I. Kinetic and cellular aspects of lymphocyte proliferative responses in diabetics. Journal of Immunology. 1983;**131**:701-705

[84] Watters C, Everett JA, Haley C, Clinton A, Rumbaugh KP. Insulin treatment modulates the host immune system to enhance *Pseudomonas aeruginosa* wound biofilms. Infection and Immunity. 2014;**82**:92-100

[85] Markgraf DF, Al-Hasani H, Lehr S. Lipidomics—Reshaping the analysis and perception of type 2 diabetes. International Journal of Molecular Sciences. 2016;**17**:1841

[86] Suvitaival T, Bondia-Pons I, Yetukuri L, Pöhö P, Nolan JJ, Hyötyläinen T, et al. Lipidome as a predictive. Tool in progression to type 2 diabetes in Finnish men. Metabolism. 2018;**78**:1-12

[87] Kopprasch S, Dheban S, Schuhmann K, Xu A, Schulte KM, Simeonovic CJ, et al. Detection of independent associations of plasma lipidomic parameters with insulin sensitivity indices using data mining methodology. PLoS One. 2016;**11**:e0164173

[88] Lydic TA, Goo Y-H. Lipidomics unveils the complexity of the lipidome in metabolic diseases. Clinical and Translational Medicine. 2018;**7**:4

Chapter 4

Dysregulation of Bile Acids in Patients with NAFLD

Xinmu Zhang and Ruitang Deng

Abstract

Bile acids are synthesized in the liver and tightly regulated through the enterohepatic circulation. Recent studies reveal that bile acids serve as hormone-like signaling molecules to activate nuclear receptors, notably farnesoid X receptor (FXR), regulating metabolic homeostasis of bile acids, cholesterol, lipids, and glucose. A connection between bile acids and nonalcoholic fatty liver disease (NAFLD) has long been recognized. Although inconsistent or even contradictory results are reported, a large body of evidence from clinical as well as preclinical studies demonstrates that bile acid homeostasis is disrupted in patients with NAFLD. The bile acid dysregulation gets worsening as NAFLD progresses from early stage simple steatosis to late stage nonalcoholic steatohepatitis (NASH) and NASH with fibrosis. As the risk factors for NAFLD, obesity and insulin resistance, which are often associated with NAFLD, contribute to the dysregulation of bile acids in patients with NAFLD. Total serum and fecal bile acid concentrations are mostly elevated in patients with NAFLD as a result of increased bile acid synthesis, elevated hepatic bile acids, and upregulation of bile acid transporters. The two negative feedback regulatory pathways for bile acid synthesis, FXR/SHP (small heterodimer partner) and fibroblast growth factor-19 (FGF19)/FGF receptor-4 (FGFR4), are impaired in patients with NAFLD.

Keywords: NAFLD, steatosis, fatty liver, NASH, bile acids, FXR, bile acid synthesis, enterohepatic circulation, bile acid transporters, FGF19

1. Introduction

Nonalcoholic fatty liver disease (NAFLD) is the most prevalent form of chronic liver disease worldwide. It affects about 30% of the population in the United States [1, 2] and 10% of adolescents and children [3, 4]. NAFLD is a spectrum of metabolic disorders starting with simple steatosis characterized with excessive accumulation of triglycerides in the hepatocytes, progressing to nonalcoholic steatohepatitis (NASH) characterized with inflammation, to fibrosis and cirrhosis, and eventually to liver failure and hepatocellular carcinoma (HCC) [5–7]. Obesity and insulin resistance or diabetes are the most prevalent risk factors for development of NAFLD [8–13].

Bile acids are the metabolites of cholesterol and synthesized in the liver. It is well known that bile acids act as biological detergents to solubilize cholesterol and lipids in the bile and intestine, play important roles in cholesterol and lipid absorption and transport. Recent studies have revealed that bile acids can serve as hormone-like signaling molecules to activate several nuclear receptors, notably the farnesoid X receptor (FXR) [14, 15]. The bile acids/FXR signaling plays critical roles in regulating a myriad of metabolic homeostasis including bile acids, cholesterol, lipids, and glucose [16–19], as well as inflammation/immunity [20–24] and liver regeneration [25–27].

Under physiological condition, bile acid homeostasis is maintained through multiple negative feedback loops for bile acid synthesis [18, 28–30] and a tightly regulated enterohepatic circulation of bile acids [31–34]. Since liver is the organ for bile acid synthesis and metabolism and biliary excretion of bile acids is the limiting step for the enterohepatic circulation [35, 36], impairment of liver function as a result of various liver disorders leads to dysregulation of bile acids. Indeed, the measurement of bile acids is considered a biomarker of liver function and serves as an indicator of hepatobiliary impairment or diseases [37–41]. On the other hand, excessive accumulation of bile acids in the liver causes liver damages by multiple mechanisms including disrupting the integrity of cell membranes through their detergent property [42–44], causing mitochondrial stress and promoting the generation of reactive oxygen species [45–48], and inducing endoplasmic reticulum stress [49–51] and inflammatory responses [52–54], resulting in cell death via apoptosis and/or necrosis [55–58].

Because of the reciprocal effects between liver damage and bile acid dysregulation, it is often difficult, if not impossible, to determine the cause-and-effect relation between liver damage and bile acid dysregulation for many liver disorders. In one hand, liver damage causes bile acid dysregulation. On the other hand, bile acid dysregulation potentially causes liver damage. The connection between NAFLD and bile acid dysregulation has long been recognized and reported [59–67]. It is well established that liver function is compromised in patients with NAFLD, especially advanced stages of NAFLD, such as NASH and NASH-associated fibrosis and cirrhosis, due to pathological and structural damages to the liver. Research interests and emphasis are recently condensed on investigating the contribution of bile acid dysregulation to the pathogenesis of NAFLD and developing therapeutic interventions for NAFLD by manipulating the bile acid signaling pathway [66–73]. However, the outcomes of clinical trials targeting bile acid signaling using ursodeoxycholic acid (UDCA) and obeticholic acid (OCA) to treat NASH patients are not very encouraging [74–79], indicating that our understanding on the relationship between bile acids and NAFLD is not complete or even may be misinterpreted.

Taken together, the link between bile acids and NAFLD has been firmly established. However, certain fundamental questions remain to be answered. How bile acid homeostasis is disrupted in patients with NAFLD? Whether dysregulation of bile acids is one of the manifestations of NAFLD or actually contributes to the development and/or progression of NAFLD? It only becomes possible to develop rationalized approaches to treat patients with NAFLD until those fundamental questions are fully addressed. In this chapter, the effects of NAFLD on bile acid homeostasis are reviewed and discussed.

2. Altered bile acid profiles in subjects with NAFLD

In human, cholic acids (CAs) and chenodeoxycholic acid (CDCA) are two primary bile acids synthesized in the liver and account for majority of bile acids in the bile acid pool. Upon excretion into intestine, primary bile acids can be converted into secondary bile acids by gut bacteria. Specifically, CA is converted into deoxycholic acid (DCA), while CDCA is converted into lithocholic acid (LCA) or UDCA in the intestine by dehydroxylation [80, 81] or 7β epimerization [82–84]. Majority of primary and secondary bile acids are conjugated by either glycine or taurine in the liver, generating glycine- or taurine-conjugated bile acids [80, 81]. Under physiological conditions, total bile acid levels, as well as the composition of the bile acid pool, are regulated and maintained. However, under various pathological conditions, especially liver disorders, the bile acid pool size or total bile acids and bile acid pool compositions are altered. A large number of clinical and preclinical studies have revealed that bile acid profiles are altered in patients with NAFLD and rodent NAFLD models.

2.1 Altered bile acid profiles in patients with NAFLD

2.1.1 Serum bile acids

Under the physiological condition, serum bile acid concentrations are much lower than those in the enterohepatic system. However, when the enterohepatic cycling of bile acids is compromised due to hepatic injuries or intestine disorders, bile acids are spilled into the blood circulation system, altering serum bile acid concentrations, as well as compositions. Bile acid profiling in healthy populations has revealed that serum bile acid concentrations and compositions are age dependent [85]. Therefore, the serum bile acid profiles in adult and children with NAFLD are separately described in the following sections.

2.1.1.1 Serum bile acid profiling in adults with NAFLD

Currently, there are total nine clinical studies investigating serum bile acid levels and compositions in adults with NAFLD. In study 1 with 25 healthy subjects, 11 patients with steatosis, and 24 patients with NASH, it was found that serum bile acid profiles after overnight fasting were significantly altered in both steatotic and NASH patients, especially in patients with NASH [86]. The most prominent alteration is the markedly increased conjugated CA concentration. Taurine-conjugated CAs (TCAs) were elevated 4- and 2.2-fold, while glycine-conjugated CAs (GCAs) were increased 4.3- and 3.1-fold in patients with NASH and steatosis, respectively. Similarly, GCDCA levels were also elevated by 2- and 2.4-fold in patients with NASH and steatosis, respectively. Other bile acid species, including CA, GDCA, TDCA, and TCDCA, exhibited a trend of increase but their levels did not reach a statistical significance. It should be noted that patients with steatosis or NASH had significantly elevated insulin levels and exhibited insulin resistance, although the blood glucose levels were within the normal range. The patients, especially those with NASH, also had elevated serum alanine aminotransferase (ALT) and aspartate aminotransferase (AST) levels, indicating liver damage in those patients.

In study 2 with 15 healthy controls and 7 NASH patients, both fasting and postprandial bile acids were altered [87]. Total fasting serum bile acid levels were increase by more than twofold. Such increases in total bile acids are mainly due to significantly increased conjugated bile acids with both glycine and taurine, while unconjugated bile acids were not significantly altered. Both primary (CDCA and CA and their conjugated) and secondary (DCA and LCA and their conjugated) bile acids were markedly elevated. Similarly, postprandial serum bile acid levels were also markedly increased in patients with NASH, including total, conjugated and unconjugated, primary, and secondary bile acids. However, the relative ratios or the compositions of the serum bile acid pools were not significantly altered in both fasting and postprandial levels. Significant elevations in individual bile acids including DCA, GCA, GCDCA, and TCA were also noted. Other bile acid species including CA and CDCA were either not altered or slightly increased without reaching a statistical significance. Patients with NASH had significantly elevated alkaline phosphatase (ALP), ALT, insulin, and homeostatic model assessment (HOMA) levels accompanied with significantly higher fast blood glucose levels when compared to the control subjects.

In study 3 with 24 healthy subjects, 25 steatotic, and 37 NASH patients, plasma bile acids after fasting were measured [88]. Total plasma primary bile acids (CA and CDCA) were gradually increased from controls to steatotic to NASH patients. On the contrary, total secondary bile acids (DCA and LCA) were gradually decreased from controls to steatotic to NASH patients. The increases in primary bile acids are mainly resulted from elevation of the conjugated bile acids, while the unconjugated primary bile acids (CA and CDCA) were comparable to those in the control subjects. Comparison between the two NAFLD groups, total conjugated CA and conjugated primary bile acids, was significantly higher in subjects with NASH compared to steatotic subjects. In addition, the compositions of the primary bile acid pools were also changed with significant increase in the ratios of total primary CA to CDCA, regardless of the status of diabetes. Although total secondary bile acids were lower in NASH patients, most of the individual secondary bile acids including GDAC, TDCA, TLCA, and GLCA were comparable among the three groups except for unconjugated DCA, which was significantly higher in NASH patients. Unconjugated UDCA levels were comparable among the three groups, while conjugated UDCA was significantly higher in NASH patients compared to steatotic and control subjects. It should be mentioned that AST and ALT levels were significantly elevated in both steatotic and NASH patients, indicating hepatic injury under the steatotic and NASH conditions. In addition, a large percentage of NASH patients (62.2%) were diabetic, while 20% of steatotic patients were diabetic with only one subject (4.2%) being diabetic in the control group.

In study 4 with 14 healthy controls and 7 patients with NASH, serum total bile acids were significantly elevated by 2.5-fold in patients with NASH compared to healthy control subjects [89]. Individual bile acids including GCA and TCA were markedly increased by 3.1- and 5.7-fold in patients with NASH, respectively. In addition, linear regression analysis revealed a significant association between NAFLD activity scores (NAS) and fasting total serum bile acid, GCA, and TCA concentrations. It should be mentioned that the fasting total bile acids, GCA and TCA serum, concentrations in healthy controls in the study were comparable to those reported previously for healthy adults [90].

In study 5 with 46 healthy control subjects and 13 patients with NAFLD, serum bile acids were dysregulated in patients with NAFLD [38]. Total serum bile acid levels were significantly increased by 4.7-fold from 2.8 μM in control subjects to 13.0 μM in NAFLD patients. Primary and secondary bile acids were elevated by 3.8- and 1.9-fold, respectively, in NAFLD patients. These increases in total, primary, and secondary bile acids are mainly due to much higher concentrations of conjugated bile acids in NAFLD patients (5.0 μM) than in control subjects (1.2 μM). Unconjugated bile acids were also slightly increased from 0.88 μM in control subjects to 1.30 μM in NAFLD patients without reaching a statistical significance.

In contrast to most of the previous studies, a recent study 6 with 32 patients with NASH and 26 non-NASH controls reported that plasma total, primary, secondary, unconjugated, and conjugated bile acids were not significantly different between the two groups [91]. The compositions of the plasma bile acid pools were also not altered either in patients with NASH when compared to non-NASH subjects. However, when the subjects were subcategorized into insulin resistance and insulin sensitive groups, significant changes in bile acid profiles were detected. Total serum CA (CA + GCA and TCA), unconjugated CA, total CDCA (CDCA + GCDCA + TCDCA), unconjugated CDCA, total primary and unconjugated primary, total unconjugated, and non-12α bile acids were all significantly elevated in subjects with insulin resistance compared to insulin sensitive subjects. The authors therefore concluded that bile acid alterations were associated with insulin resistance but not NASH. The study also showed that body mass index (BMI), fasting plasma insulin concentrations, and HOMA values positively correlated with plasma CA and CDCA levels. It should be mentioned that the BMI and HOMA values were matched between the NASH patients and the non-NASH control subjects in this study. The average BMI was 40.2 for NASH and 39.4 for non-Nash subjects, indicating that both groups are severely obese. The average HOMA was 4.05 for NASH patients and 3.25 for non-NASH controls, indicating insulin resistance in both groups.

Consistent with the findings from the sixth study, another clinical study reported that patients with NAFLD exhibited comparable serum total bile acid concentrations to those in healthy control subjects [92]. The study included 16 healthy controls with an average BMI of 24.2, 14 overweight NAFLD patients with BMI of 28.3, and 12 obese NAFLD patients with an average BMI of 35.3. No significant alterations in fasting as well as postprandial serum total bile acid levels were detected between healthy control subjects and overweight or obese NAFLD patients.

In another study with 38 control subjects and 36 NASH patients, limited information about the characteristics of the studied subjects was provided and only data on three individual bile acid species were reported. The plasma concentrations of GCA, TCA, and TCDCA during fasting were significantly elevated in patients with NASH compared to control subjects [93]. Consistent with finding from most of the studies, another clinical study with 10 healthy controls, 39 steatotic, and 59 NASH patients reported that total serum bile acid levels were significantly elevated in patients with NAFLD [94].

The findings from six clinical studies, which provide detailed characteristics of the studied subjects as well as the corresponding bile acid profiles, are summarized in **Table 1**. The results from studies 1 to 5 are largely consistent. Serum total, primary, and conjugated bile acids were all significantly increased with limited changes for unconjugated bile acids. However, the secondary bile acids were significantly increased in studies 1, 2, and 5 but decreased in study 3. In contrast to the findings from studies 1 to 5, no significant alterations were detected in serum total, primary, secondary, conjugated, and unconjugated bile acids in the study 6.

Compared the characteristics of the control and NAFLD subjects, it is noticed that the control subjects in study 6 were severely obese with BMI 39.4 ± 5.9, while the control subjects in studies 1–5 have normal or close to normal body weights with BMI ranging from 24.5 ± 2.6 to 27.3 ± 5.8. The BMI values were matched between NAFLD patients and control subjects in study 6 but significantly different in studies 1–5. Compared with serum bile acid levels in a healthy population [85], the control subjects in study 6 had markedly increased total, primary, secondary, conjugated, and unconjugated bile acids. The results indicate that obesity or increased BMI is a contributing factor to the dysregulation of serum bile acids. Indeed, several studies have reported that subjects with overweight or obese had increased serum bile acid concentrations [85, 95, 96].

The second characteristic of the studied subjects that is different between study 6 and studies 1–5 is the status of insulin resistance in the control subjects. The serum insulin levels and HOMA values in study 6 are markedly higher than those in the other five studies, suggesting that insulin resistance is a contributing factor for the dysregulation of serum bile acids. Indeed, when all the subjects (NAFLD and control patients) in the study 6 were separated by insulin resistance status, primary bile acids, unconjugated bile acids, and non-12α bile acids, total CA and total CDCA were significantly increased in subjects with

Features	Subjects	Study 1 [87]	Study 2 [88]	Study 3 [89]	Study 4 [90]	Study 5 [92]	Study 6 [93]
Sample size	Control	25	15	24	14	46	26
	Steatosis	11		25			
	NASH	24	7	37	7	13	32
Age	Control	42.6 ± 9.2	43 ± 12	39.2 ± 12.4	42 ± 13	20–39	40.5 ± 11.7
	Steatosis	43.5 ± 10.7		54.6 ± 10.1			
	NASH	43.6 ± 12.6	48 ± 10	58.0 ± 8.8	48 ± 10	62.5 ± 16.5	41.3 ± 11.9
BMI	Control	24.5 ± 2.6	25 ± 2.7	27.3 ± 5.8	26 ± 2.7	<25	39.4 ± 5.9
	Steatosis	34.0 ± 4.0		32.6 ± 5.4			
	NASH	34.8 ± 4.7	32.0 ± 5.2	34.4 ± 4.2	32 ± 5.2	25.5 ± 2.8	40.2 ± 5.8
Insulin	Control	7.6 ± 3.1	7.6 ± 2.6	N/A	8.0 ± 3.0	N/A	15.7 ± 9.1
	Steatosis	20.6 ± 9.0		N/A			
	NASH	26.5 ± 14.9	40 ± 27	N/A	40 ± 27	N/A	18.9 ± 11.4
HOMA-IR	Control	0.9 ± 0.4	1.6 ± 0.6	1 (4.2%) diabetic	2.0 ± 1.0	0% DM	3.25 ± 2.05
	Steatosis	2.6 ± 1.1		5 (20%) diabetic			
	NASH	3.26 ± 1.6	13 ± 8.7	23 (62%) diabetic	12 ± 9.0	53.8% DM	4.05 ± 2.65
ALT	Control	17.6 ± 5.0	33 ± 11	22.7 ± 15.5	33 ± 11	Normal	27.3 ± 15.8
	Steatosis	44.4 ± 30.0		45.5 ± 24.0			
	NASH	84.6 ± 58.6	75 ± 36	57.1 ± 29.3	75 ± 36	64.1 (34.2–120)	36.5 ± 22.7
AST	Control	22.8 ± 5.7	N/A	22.3 ± 11.3	N/A	Normal	21.3 ± 11.9
	Steatosis	31.4 ± 15.4		45.6 ± 51.9			
	NASH	63.4 ± 46.7	N/A	42.4 ± 18.7	N/A	46.2 (26.8–79.8)	24.6 ± 17.5
Bile acids	Total	Increased	Increased	Increased	Increased	Increased	No changes
	Primary	Increased	Increased	Increased	Increased	Increased	No changes
	Secondary	Increased	Increased	Decreased	N/A	Increased	No changes
	Conjugated	Increased	Increased	Increased	Increased	Increased	No changes
	Unconjugated	N/A*	Increased but not significant	No changes	N/A	Slightly increased	No changes
	Compositions of bile acids	N/A	No significant changes	Significantly altered	N/A	N/A	No changes

**N/A, not available.*

Table 1.
Dysregulation of bile acids in adults with NAFLD with characteristics of the studied subjects.

insulin resistance compared to insulin sensitive subjects regardless of the status of NAFLD. These data strongly suggest that insulin resistance is a contributing factor to the dysregulation of bile acids, which is supported by the findings from previous studies [95–100].

The third different characteristic of the NASH patients in study 6 from studies 1 to 5 is the liver injury status. The NASH patients in study 6 exhibited much lower ALT and AST levels than those in the NASH patients in studies 1–5, indicating that the NASH patients in study 6 experienced minimal liver injury, while the NASH patients in other studies exhibited hepatic injury or damage with the ALT and AST levels above the physiological values. As discussed earlier, it is well established that liver injury potentially can cause dysregulation of bile acids [38–42]. The differing liver injury statuses may provide an explanation for the discrepancy in bile acid alterations between the study 6 and the other five studies. Taken together, the characteristic variations in BMI, insulin resistance, and hepatic injury of the studied subjects may all contribute to the inconsistency in serum bile acid levels reported in those studies.

2.1.1.2 Serum bile acid profiling in children with NAFLD

There are three studies conducted with children from ages 4 to 17 years old. In one study with 11 healthy controls (average age 12.8 years) and 16 patients with NASH (average age 13.7 years), total serum bile acid levels were significantly elevated by threefold in children with NASH compared to healthy controls [101]. More specifically, the absolute concentrations of CA, CDCA, DCA, and UDCA were all markedly increased. The percentages of CA and DCA in the total bile acid pools were significantly increased, while the percentages of CDCA in the pools were decreased with no changes in UDCA. It is noted that both ALT and AST levels in patients with NASH were increased, indicating hepatic injury in those patients. The children with NASH also exhibited insulin resistance with an average HOMA value of 4.3 ± 2.8 and overweight or obese with an average BMI of 33.8 ± 7.7.

In the second study with 105 healthy controls at ages 9.3 ± 2.5 and 92 children with NAFLD, which were further classified into two groups based on the stages of fibrosis: NAFLD-F0 group at ages 10.9 ± 3.7 and F ≥ 1 group at ages 11.5 ± 1.9, total serum bile acids were significantly decreased from 3.6 μM in control subjects to 1.73 μM in nonfibrotic (NAFLD-F0) patients accompanied by decreased glycine-conjugated bile acids and slightly increased taurine-conjugated and unconjugated bile acids [102]. The total serum bile acids in patients with more advanced NAFLD with fibrosis (NAFLD-F ≥ 1) were also decreased to 2.45 μM. Comparison between the two NAFLD groups, the serum bile acid levels increased by 41.9% in the NAFLD-F ≥ 1 group. These data indicate that serum bile acid levels decrease in the early stage of NAFLD, followed by an increase as NAFLD progresses to fibrosis. No significant differences were detected in the compositions of serum total bile acid pools among the groups. It should be mentioned that compared with control subjects (BMI 18.8 ± 4.2), children in the NAFLD groups were overweight (BMI > 26) with significantly elevated glucose and insulin levels. In addition, NAFLD patients had elevated AST and ALT levels, indicating hepatic injury in those patients.

In a most recent third study with 35 control children at ages 12.8 ± 4.2 and 41 NAFLD children at ages 13.7 ± 2.4, which were further divided into mild and moderate/severe NAFLD groups, no significant alternations in serum total, primary, and secondary bile acids were detected in children with NAFLD compared to control subjects [103]. Most of individual bile acid species (CA, CDCA, DCA, and LCA), conjugated and unconjugated bile acids, were comparable among the groups. Significant differences were only detected for unconjugated CDCA and unconjugated primary bile acids (CDCA + CA). Unconjugated CDCA and primary bile acids increased by 1.58-fold and 1.43-fold, respectively, in NAFLD children. After adjusted for age, sex, HOMA and BMI, unconjugated DCA, conjugated DCA

(GDCA and TDCA), and total DCA were significantly lower in NAFLD patients than those in the control group. Meanwhile, serum GLCA and total conjugated LCA (GCA + TLCA) were significantly decreased in NAFLD patients compared to control subjects.

The findings from the three clinical studies with detailed characteristics of the studied subjects are summarized in **Table 2**. The results from the three studies are largely inconsistent. In the second study with a larger size of samples, serum bile acid levels decrease in early stage of NAFLD and then increase during progression to fibrosis, but the levels were still below that in control subjects. In the third study with a medium size of samples, no significant alternations in serum total, primary, and secondary bile acids were detected in children with NAFLD. However, in the first study with smallest size of samples, total serum bile acid levels and compositions were significantly altered in patients with NASH compared to healthy controls.

Comparing the characteristics of studied subjects, the trend of bile acid alterations from decrease to no changes to increase correlates with the trend of gradually increased BMI from slightly overweight (26.5 ± 3.59) to severe overweight (29.6 ± 5.2) to obese (33.8 ± 7.7). Such correlation indicates that NAFLD-associated overweight or obesity may play important roles in influencing the bile acid homeostasis in children as well [85, 95, 96]. Another possible factor playing a role in bile acid dysregulation under the NAFLD conditions is the HOMA values, which were increased from 3.0 ± 3.0 in study 1 to 4.1 ± 3.2 in study 2 and 4.3 ± 2.8 in study 3. The differences in sample sizes of the studies certainly also contribute to the variations of bile acid levels among the studies. The sample sizes in the control groups ranged from 105 in study 2 to 35 in study 3 to 11 in study 1. Meanwhile, the sample sizes for NAFLD subjects were decreased from 92 in study 2 to 42 in study 3 to 16 in study 1. Taken together, serum bile acid levels were differentially altered in children with NAFLD. The differences in BMI, insulin resistance, and sample sizes may contribute to the variations of serum bile acids detected among the three studies.

2.1.2 Hepatic bile acids

There are three relevant studies investigating hepatic bile acids in patients with NAFLD. In the first study with 15 NASH patients and 8 control subjects, total hepatic bile acids were significantly increased in patients with NASH compared to control subjects [104]. The concentrations of individual bile acid species including CA, CDCA, and DCA were markedly higher in patients with NASH than those in the controls. It was also found that hepatic total bile acid levels were significantly correlated with hepatic inflammation status. Meanwhile, CDCA concentrations were positively correlated with fibrosis status in patients with NASH.

In a second study with liver tissues from 17 normal control subjects, 4 patients with simple steatosis, and 37 patients with NASH, significant alterations in hepatic bile acids were detected in NASH patients [105]. Hepatic CA and GDCA concentrations were markedly decreased by 69 and 91%, respectively, in patients with NASH compared to the control subjects. In contrast, hepatic TCA, TDCA, and GCDCA were significantly increased by approximately three, five, and twofold in NASH patients, respectively. Overall, hepatic total and conjugated bile acid concentrations were significantly higher in patients with NASH than those in controls. On the other hand, unconjugated bile acids were significantly decreased in patients with NASH. In patients with simple steatosis, total, conjugated, and unconjugated bile acids were all decreased without reaching a statistical significance mainly due to a small sample size of the group.

Features	Subjects	Study 1 [104]	Study 2 [105]	Study 3 [106]
Sample size	Control	11	105	35
	Steatosis		27	18
	NASH	16	65	23
Age	Control	12.8 ± 4.2	16 ± 3	9.3 ± 2.5
	Steatosis		10 ± 5	10.9 ± 3.7
	NASH	13.7 ± 2.4	12 ± 5	11.5 ± 1.9
BMI	Control	19.2 ± 3.4	20.5 ± 4.2	18.8 ± 4.2
	Steatosis		26.8 ± 3.9	26.0 ± 5.1
	NASH	33.8 ± 7.7	26.5 ± 3.5	29.6 ± 5.2
Insulin	Control	N/A*	3.2 ± 0.6	6.9 ± 4.9
	Steatosis		11.2 ± 4.8	11.0 ± 5.9
	NASH	N/A	12.4 ± 6.0	17.5 ± 11.4
HOMA-IR	Control	N/A	1.5 ± 0.3	1.3 ± 1.0
	Steatosis		2.6 ± 1.8	2.6 ± 1.5
	NASH	4.3 ± 2.8	3.0 ± 3.0	4.1 ± 3.2
ALT	Control	19.4 ± 4.4	24 ± 28	14.0 ± 8.5
	Steatosis		62 ± 20	25.5 ± 17
	NASH	54.1 ± 29.7	87 ± 59	68.5 ± 42.0
AST	Control	24.4 ± 11.5	25 ± 13	25 ± 8.5
	Steatosis		40 ± 8	23 ± 6.7
	NASH	33.9 ± 15.0	61 ± 29	40.9 ± 24.7
Bile acids	Total	Significantly increased	Significantly decreased	No significant changes
	Primary	Significantly increased	Significantly decreased	No significant changes
	Secondary	Significantly increased	Slightly decreased	No significant changes
	Conjugated	N/A	Significantly decreased	No significant changes
	Unconjugated	N/A	Slightly increased	No significant changes
	Compositions of bile acids	Significantly altered	No changes	No changes

**N/A, not available.*

Table 2.
Dysregulation of bile acids in children with NAFLD with characteristics of the studied subjects.

In a relevant third study with 20 control subjects and 22 diabetic patients, hepatic bile acid concentrations were significantly altered [106]. Among the 22 diabetic patients, 77.7% patients had NAFLD with NAS score of 2 or above. Consistently, majority of patients (68%) were overweight, obese, or severe obese, with hypercholesterolemia being detected in 86.4% of the patients. Total hepatic bile acids were markedly reduced by 53% in diabetic patients compared to control subjects. The significant decrease in total bile acids is largely due to the marked reduction in conjugated bile acids. On the other hand, unconjugated bile acids were slightly increased by 33% without reaching a statistical significance. Among the conjugated bile acids, both glycine and taurine conjugated bile acids were significantly reduced in diabetic patients. However, the reductions were more severe in glycine conjugated than taurine-conjugated bile acids.

In summary, no clear consensus can be reached for hepatic bile acid profiles in patients with NAFLD. Both increases and decreases of hepatic bile acids were reported. Some specific bile acid species were markedly increased, while other species significantly decreased in the same patients. From the limited clinical studies, it can be concluded that hepatic bile acid homeostasis is dysregulated in patients with NAFLD. However, due to the complexity of bile acid regulation, variations in characteristics and stages of NAFLD patients, and lack of high quality clinical studies, it largely remains to be determined by the effects of NAFLD on hepatic bile acid homeostasis.

2.1.3 Fecal and urine bile acids

There are only one study investigating fecal bile acids in patients with NAFLD. The study has 25 healthy controls, 12 patients with steatosis, and 17 patients with NASH [107]. Total fecal bile acid levels were significantly higher in patients with NASH compared to healthy controls. Meanwhile, total fecal bile acids also showed an increased trend in steatotic patients without reaching a statistical significance. Primary, secondary, conjugated, and unconjugated bile acid concentrations all exhibited a gradual increase from healthy controls to steatotic to NASH patients. Unconjugated primary bile acids including CA and CDCA were significantly increased in NASH patients compared to healthy controls, while unconjugated secondary bile acids were not significantly different among the three groups. Patients with NASH had significantly higher concentrations of conjugated LCA compared to patients with steatosis. In addition, a higher ratio of primary to secondary bile acids in patients with NASH was also detected. However, the ratio of total conjugated over unconjugated bile acids was not significantly different among the groups. Correlation analysis revealed that fecal unconjugated primary bile acids positively correlated with steatosis, ballooning, fibrosis, NAS scores, and liver injury (AST and ALT levels). The results from the study demonstrated that fecal disposition of bile acids was enhanced in patients with NASH. However, it remains to be determined that such increase in fecal disposition of bile acids is resulted from impairment of intestine reabsorption of bile acids or enhanced biliary excretion of bile acids or both.

There is only one study with 15 healthy controls and 7 NASH patients to investigate urine bile acid profiles in patients with NAFLD. Urine total, primary, secondary, conjugated, and unconjugated bile acids all exhibited a trend of increase without reaching a statistical significance [87]. However, individual bile acid species including DCA, TCA, GCA, and GCDCA were significantly elevated in patients with NASH compared to control subjects. Consistently, total serum bile acid levels were also significantly increased by more than twofold in NASH patients compared to control subjects.

In summary, the findings from clinical studies to evaluate serum, hepatic, and urine bile acid profiles are inconsistent among the studies. The reasons for those inconsistent or even conflicting results are multiple folds. First, bile acid synthesis and serum concentrations fluctuate during the days and nights [108–112].

Although most of the samples were collected after fasting, there was no mentioning on exactly when the samples were collected in the studies. Second, NAFLD represents a spectrum of pathological liver conditions from simple steatosis to NASH with or without fibrosis. The severity of bile acid dysregulation appears NAFLD stage dependent. Bile acid alterations gets worsening in patients with advanced stages of NAFLD, such as NASH, compared to the patients with simple steatosis [86, 88, 101, 102, 107]. Some studies differentiate NAFLD patients into simple steatosis and NASH [86, 88, 101, 102, 107], while the others [38, 87, 89, 91, 103] do not, which certainly influences the outcomes of the studies. Third, NAFLD is often associated with various metabolic conditions, especially obesity and insulin resistance/diabetes. It has been reported that obesity and insulin resistance directly impacts bile acid homeostasis [85, 95–100]. Fourth, selection of the control groups varies from study to study [38, 86–89, 91], which certainly contributes to the discrepancy of the outcomes among the studies. Finally, the sizes of samples are relatively small in most of the studies with individual variations potentially masking the alterations.

2.2 Altered bile acid profiles in NAFLD animal models

Several rodent models for NAFLD have been developed [113–115], including high-fat cholesterol (HFC) and methionine- and choline-deficient (MCD) diet-induced or genetic deficient models, including leptin-deficient *ob/ob*, leptin receptor-deficient *db/db* mice, and *fa/fa* rats. Several preclinical studies were conducted to investigate the effects of NAFLD on bile acid homeostasis using NAFLD mouse or rat models. In one study, NAFLD was induced in rats with HFC diet [116]. Total hepatic bile acids were significantly increased in rats on HFC diet for 2 weeks. Primary, secondary, conjugated, and unconjugated bile acid concentrations were all increased after 2 weeks on HFC diet. Most bile acid species remained higher in rats on HFC diet for 8 and 14 weeks than those on regular diet. However, the levels of CA and DCA species declined from their peaks at 2 weeks, while CDCA species persistently increased for the entire treatment. In addition, CDCA species positively correlated with macrovesicular steatosis score, serum ALT levels, and quantified fibrotic area. Among the conjugated bile acids, glycine-conjugated bile acid species (GCA, GCDCA, GDCA, GLCA, and GUDCA) were predominate over taurine-conjugated bile acid species and positively correlated with macrovesicular steatosis score. The finding demonstrated that bile acid homeostasis is severely disrupted in HFC diet-induced NAFLD rats, especially the CDCA and glycine-conjugated bile acid species.

In another study with MCD-induced NASH mouse model, markedly increased serum concentrations of taurine-conjugated CA and β-muricholate (βMCA) were detected in mice on MCD diet for 2 or 8 weeks compared to mice on control diet, indicating dysregulation of serum bile acid in mice with NASH [117]. Similar findings were reported with *ob/ob* mouse model. Serum total bile acid concentrations were markedly elevated by sevenfold from 1.9 ± 1.0 μM in wt control mice to 14.9 ± 5.4 μM in *ob/ob* mice [118]. In contrast to the findings from the studies described above, a more recent study showed that total serum bile acid concentrations were not significantly different in HFD-induced NAFLD mice than mice on control diet [119].

Taken together, bile acid homeostasis is disrupted in NAFLD rodent models. Serum bile acid levels were markedly elevated in most of the studies. However, variations in serum bile acid concentrations exist in different NAFLD rodent models, may reflecting species difference between mouse and rat.

3. Alterations in bile acid synthesis in subjects with NAFLD

3.1 Alterations in bile acid synthesis in patients with NAFLD

Primary bile acids CA and CDCA are synthesized in the liver through either the classical or alternative synthesis pathways. In the intestine, CA can be converted into secondary bile acid DCA, while CDCA is converted into secondary bile acids LCA or UDCA (**Figure 1**). Cholesterol 7α-hydroxylase (CYP7A1) is the rate-limiting enzyme in the classical pathway, while CYP8B1 is the rate-limiting enzyme for the production of CA. The two rate-limiting enzymes for the alternative pathway are CYP27A1 and CYP7B1 (**Figure 1**). Alterations in the expression levels of rate-limiting enzymes in the bile acid synthesis pathways result in dysregulation of bile acid homeostasis. A number of clinical studies have conducted to investigate the effects of NAFLD on bile acid synthesis.

3.1.1 CYP7A1

There are eight clinical studies investigating the expression of CYP7A1 in patients with NAFLD. Most of the studies revealed that CYP7A1 expression was dysregulated in patients with NAFLD. Among the eight studies, the results from five studies showed that the mRNA expression levels of CYP7A1 were significantly increased in patients with NAFLD [88, 91, 94, 101, 120], indicating that bile acid synthesis through the classical pathway is enhanced in patients with NAFLD. However, in a study with 17 normal control subjects, 4 patients with simple steatosis, and 37 patients with NASH, CYP7A1 expression was not altered in patients with steatosis or NASH [105]. In another study with 6 lean healthy controls, 20 obese normal controls, 20 patients with simple steatosis, and 20 patients with NASH [121], CYP7A1 mRNA expression significantly increased in obese normal control subjects, patients with steatosis, and NASH compared to healthy lean subjects. However, at the protein level, CYP7A1 expression was comparable in obese normal controls compared to healthy lean subjects. More

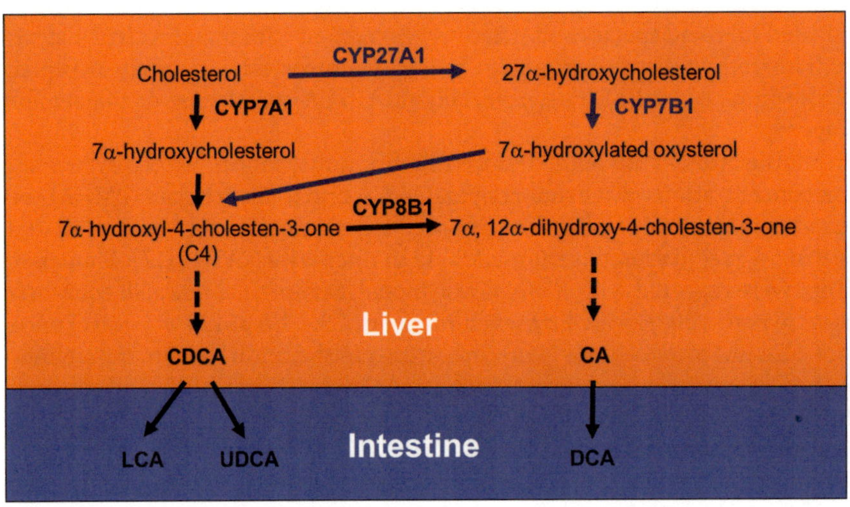

Figure 1.
Primary bile acids CDCA and CA are synthesized in the liver through classical (CYP7A1) and alternative (CYP27A1) bile acid synthesis pathways and converted into secondary bile acids LCA, UDCA, and DCA in the intestine.

strikingly, CYP7A1 protein expression was markedly decreased in patients with steatosis and especially with NASH, indicating that bile acid synthesis through the classical pathway is reduced in patients with NAFLD. In a study with 78 NAFLD patients, the subjects were divided into three groups based on the NAS scores, NAS 1–2, NAS 3–4, and NAS 5–8. The mRNA expression levels of CYP7A1 were comparable among the three groups, indicating that bile acid synthesis through the classical pathway remains unchanged during the progression of NAFLD [122].

Taken together, CYP7A1 expression was largely upregulated in patients with NAFLD, indicating that bile acid synthesis through the classical pathway is enhanced in patients with NAFLD. Discrepancy in CYP7A1 mRNA and protein levels was noted, indicating the importance of post-transcriptional regulation of CYP7A1 under the NAFLD condition.

3.1.2 CYP27A1

There are three clinical studies evaluating the effects of NAFLD on the expression of CYP27A1. The findings from the three studies are largely inconsistent. In one study, the expression levels of CYP27A1 were significantly induced in patients with NAFLD [101]. In contrast, a second study reported that CYP27A1 expression was significantly decreased in patients with NAFLD compared to control subjects [105]. A third study showed that CYP27A1 expression was not altered in NAFLD subjects [121]. Therefore, it can be concluded that the effects of NAFLD on CYP27A1 expression are inclusive.

3.1.3 Other enzymes

There are a couple of studies investigating other enzymes involved in bile acid synthesis, including CYP8B1 and CYP7B1. One study reported that the expression levels of CYP8B1 were decreased, while CYP7B1 levels were increased in patients with NAFLD [105]. The other study revealed that the expression levels of CYP8B1 were significantly increased in patients with NAFLD compared to control subjects [101]. Therefore, additional studies are required to determine the effects of NAFLD on CYP8B1 and CYP7B1 expression.

3.1.4 C4

7α-Hydroxy-4-cholesten-3-one (C4) is an intermediate of bile acid synthesis (**Figure 1**) and serves as an indicator for bile acid synthesis *in vivo* [123]. There are three studies investigating serum C4 levels in patients with NAFLD. In one study with 26 NAFLD patients and 16 healthy controls, the serum concentrations of C4 were not significantly different between the two groups, indicating that de novel bile acid synthesis was not changed in patients with NAFLD [38]. Consistent results were obtained with a second study which includes 26 healthy controls and 32 patients with NASH. The serum C4 concentrations were not significantly altered in patients with NASH compared to the control subjects [90]. However, in the third study with 25 healthy controls, 12 patients with steatosis, and 16 patients with NASH, serum C4 levels were significantly elevated in patients with steatosis and NASH compared to healthy control subjects, suggesting that bile acid synthesis is enhanced in patients with NAFLD. Correlation analysis revealed that the serum C4 concentrations were directly correlated with fecal total bile acid levels in the studied subjects [104]. Taken together, the serum C4 concentrations either increased or did not change in patients with NAFLD.

3.2 Alterations in bile acid synthesis in NAFLD animal models

There are five studies investigating the expression of enzymes involved in bile acid synthesis. In one study with high fat diet (HFD)–induced NAFLD mice, the mRNA expression levels of Cyp7a1 and Cyp8b1 were markedly decreased compared to control mice on regular diet [124], indicating that de novel bile acid synthesis through the classical pathway is reduced in NAFLD mice. Consistent with the finding, a study with *ob/ob* mice, the expression levels of Cyp7a1 were significantly decreased in *ob/ob* mice compared to lean wt mice [118]. However, in a study with HFD/streptozotocin (STZ)-induced NAFLD rats, the expression levels of Cyp7a1 were dramatically increased, while the expression levels of Cyp27a1 and Cyp7b1 were also significantly induced in NAFLD rats compared to control rats [125]. The findings indicate that bile acid synthesis through both classical and alternative pathway is increased in HFD/STZ-induced NAFLD rats. On the other hand, in one study with MCD-induced simple steatotic rats, the expression levels of Cyp7a1 were comparable between the steatotic rats and healthy control rats [126]. Consistently, a study with MCD-induced NASH in mice showed that the expression levels of Cyp7a1 were not altered in mice with NASH compared to control mice [117]. In addition, the expression levels of Cyp27a1 and Cyp8b1 were not significantly changed in steatotic mice compared to healthy control mice. The findings indicate that both classical and alternative bile acid synthesis pathways are not impaired in MCD-induced NASH mice. In summary, the effects of NAFLD on Cyp7a1, Cyp27a1, and Cyp8b1 expression are inconclusive in NAFLD rodent models, which are to a large extent different from the findings in patients with NAFLD, especially for CYP7A1.

4. Alterations in bile acid transporters in subjects with NAFLD

The enterohepatic circulation of bile acids is mediated by a series of bile acid transporters in the liver and intestine (**Figure 2**). After synthesis in the liver, bile acids are excreted into bile through the bile salt export pump (BSEP). Majority of bile acids are actively transported into enterocytes by the apical sodium-dependent bile acid transporter (ASBT). Bile acids exit the enterocytes on the basolateral side via the heterodimeric organic solute transporter α and β (OSTα/β) and then return to the liver through the Na^+/taurocholate cotransporting polypeptide (NTCP), completing the circulation. In the liver, other transporters are also capable of transport bile acids, including multidrug resistance associated protein 2 (MRP2) on the canalicular membrane and multidrug resistance-associated protein 3 (MRP3), MRP4, and organic anion-transporting polypeptides (OATP1B1 and OATP1B3) on the basolateral membrane. It should be emphasized that biliary excretion through BSEP is the rate-limiting step in the circulation and bile acid spilling into blood is mediated mainly by MRP3 and MRP4. Alteration in bile acid transporter expression has significant impact on bile acid compartmenting and homeostasis.

4.1 Alterations in bile acid transporters in patients with NAFLD

4.1.1 BSEP

As the canalicular bile acid transporter, BSEP expression was dysregulated in patients with NAFLD. Three clinical studies showed that BSEP mRNA expression

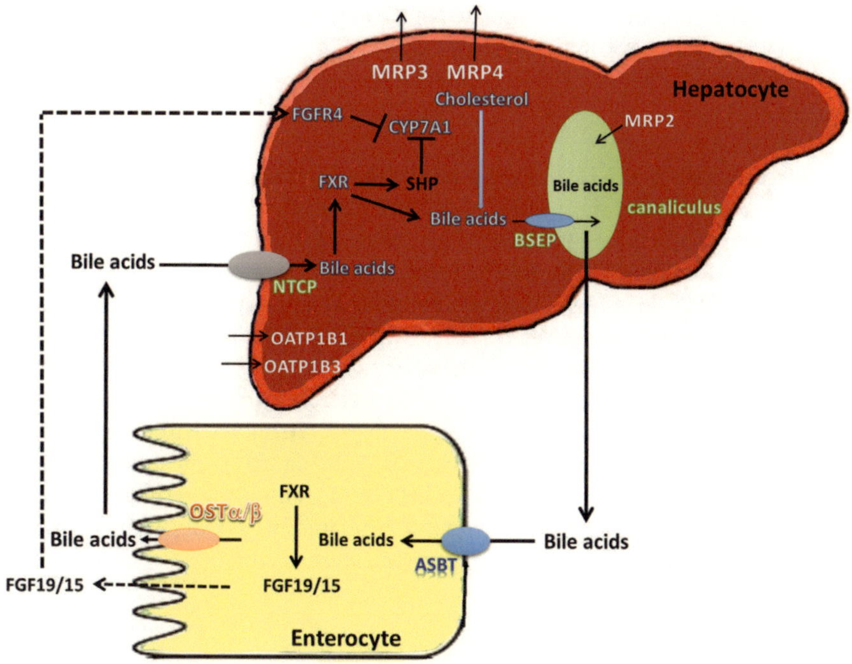

Figure 2.
Enterohepatic circulation of bile acids through a series of bile acid transporters, and regulation of bile acid synthesis by the FXR/SHP and FGF19/FGFR4 synthesis pathway.

was decreased in steatotic or NASH patients compared to control subjects [88, 91, 122]. A different study reported that BSEP mRNA expression levels were increased in patients with NASH compared to the patients with simple steatosis [118]. On the other hand, two studies revealed that BSEP mRNA expression was not altered in patients with NAFLD or diabetes compared to healthy control subjects [101, 106]. Finally, another study reported that BSEP mRNA levels were elevated in lean NAFLD patients but reduced in overweight or obese patients with steatosis or NASH [94], indicating that body weight of the patients influences the expression of BSEP under the NAFLD condition. Taken together, it can be cautiously concluded that BSEP expression was largely decreased in patients with NAFLD. The alterations BSEP expression may be influenced by the body weight of the patients.

4.1.2 NTCP

Three clinical studies showed that NTCP mRNA expression levels were significantly upregulated in patients with NAFLD compared to control subjects [88, 101, 94]. However, a different study reported that NTCP mRNA expression was significantly decreased as NAFLD progressed from earlier stage (steatosis) to late stage (NASH) [122]. On the other hand, one study reported that the mRNA levels of NTCP were significantly increased in patients with NASH compared to patients with simple steatosis. However, at the protein level, NTCP expression was significantly reduced in the patients with NASH compared to patients with simple steatosis [127], indicating the dominance of post-transcriptional regulation of NTCP under the NASH condition. Another study with diabetic patients reported that NTCP mRNA expression levels were comparable between diabetic patients and control subjects [106]. In summary, NTCP expression was likely upregulated in NAFLD patients with certain inconsistency.

4.1.3 MRPs

In one study with NAFLD and one study with diabetic patients, MRP2 mRNA expression levels were not significantly altered in NAFLD and diabetic patients compared to control subjects [88, 106]. Another study reported that MRP2 mRNA expression levels were decreased as the NAFLD progressed from steatosis to NASH [122]. Supporting MRP2's role in NAFLD, it was found that a polymorphism in MRP2 was significantly associated with NAFLD [128]. Currently, there is only one study investigating the expression levels of MRP3 in patients with NAFLD. The MRP3 mRNA expression levels were significantly elevated in patients with NAFLD, especially with NASH, compared to the healthy control subjects [94]. In another study with diabetic patients, MRP3 and MRP4 expression levels were not significantly altered in diabetic patients compared to control subjects [106]. Taken together, the results from limited studies suggest that MRP3 and MRP4 were upregulated in patients with NAFLD, while the effects of NAFLD on MRP2 expression were minimal.

4.1.4 OATPs

There is currently only one study investigating the expression of OATPs in patients with NAFLD. Both OATP1B1 and OATP1B3 mRNA expression levels were significantly upregulated in patients with NAFLD compared to control subjects [101]. In a different study with diabetic patients, the expression levels of OATP1B1 were comparable in diabetic patients compared to control subjects [106]. Therefore, it can be cautiously concluded that OATP1B1 and OATP1b3 expression were largely induced in patients with NAFLD.

4.2 Alterations in bile acid transporters in NAFLD animal models

4.2.1 Bsep

Several studies have investigated the effects of NAFLD on Bsep expression in rodents. In one study with HFD/STZ-induced NAFLD rats, the Bsep mRNA levels were significantly downregulated in NAFLD rats compared to control rats [125], indicating reducing biliary excretion of bile acids in HFD/STZ-induced NAFLD rats. However, in two other studies with MCD-induced NAFLD rats and mice, the mRNA expression levels of Bsep were not altered in NAFLD rats or mice [126, 117]. Consistently, a study with obese zucker rats showed that Bsep expression was not significantly altered in obese ZR rats compared to control rats [129]. In another study with obese ZR rats, the expression levels of Bsep mRNA were significantly decreased in obese ZR rats, while Bsep protein levels detected by Western blot as well as immunohistochemistry were comparable between obese ZR rats and lean control rats [130]. In another study with *ob/ob* mice, the expression levels of Bsep mRNA were significantly increased in *ob/ob* mice compared to lean control mice. However, in contrast to the mRNA levels, Bsep protein levels were significantly decreased in *ob/ob* mice when compared to lean control mice [118]. Consistent with decreased Bsep expression in NAFLD mice, overexpression of Bsep increases hepatobiliary lipid secretion and reduces hepatic steatosis [131]. Taken together, Bsep expression was either not altered or decreased in NAFLD rodent models.

4.2.2 Ntcp

Currently, there are six studies evaluating the effects of NAFLD on Ntcp expression in rodents. In three studies, the expression levels of Ntcp were consistently decreased in animals with NAFLD compared to control animals [117, 125, 132]. Two studies were conducted in rats, while one study was carried out in mice. The common feature among the three studies is that NAFLD was induced by MCD for 8 weeks. In the same study [132], Ntcp expression levels were also significantly decreased when NAFLD was induced by HFD. On the other hand, another two studies with rats showed the Ntcp expression was not altered under the NAFLD condition [126, 130]. Different effects of NAFLD on Ntcp mRNA and protein expression were reported in a study with *ob/ob* mice [118]. The expression levels of Ntcp mRNA were not changed in *ob/ob* mice compared to the lean control mice. However, Ntcp protein levels were significantly lower in *ob/ob* mice than those in lean control mice. Taken together, the effects of NAFLD on Ntcp expression were largely consistent among the six studies, either no significant changes or decreased dependent on the species and methods by which NAFLD was induced.

4.2.3 Mrps

The effects of NAFLD on Mrp expression were extensively investigated mainly due to the fact that Mrps are important transporters for xenobiotics including drugs. Data from eight studies evaluating Mrp2 expression in NAFLD rodents are not consistent. Two studies with obese ZR rats reported consistent results that the expression levels of Mrp2 mRNA and protein were significantly downregulated in obese ZR rats compared to lean control rats [129, 130]. Consistent with downregulation of Mrp2 in obese zucker rats, Mrp2 expression levels were reduced in MCD-induced NAFLD rats compared to control rats on supplemented MCD [126]. On the other hand, other two studies showed that Mrp2 expression levels were not significantly altered in MCD-induced NAFLD rats or HFD/STZ-induced NAFLD mice compared to the control rats or mice [117, 125]. In a study with *ob/ob* mice, Mrp2 expression levels were significantly increased at the mRNA level but decreased at the protein level [118]. In contrast, the mRNA levels of Mrp2 were decreased but protein levels were increased in MCD-induced NAFLD rats [132]. In a comprehensive study to evaluate various NAFLD models with mice and rats, Mrp2 expression was significantly increased in athrogenic diet and MCD-induced NAFLD rats and all four types of NAFLD mouse models when compared to the corresponding control rats or mice. At the protein level, Mrp2 expression was only increased in MCD-induced NAFLD rats [133]. Compared with Mrp2, the data for the effects of NAFLD on the expression of Mrp3 and Mrp4 are more consistent among the studies. Mrp3 and/or Mrp4 expression were significantly upregulated in five studies with NAFLD rats or mice [117, 124, 126, 118, 133]. On the other hand, another three studies with HFD/STZ-induced NAFLD rats or obese ZR rats reported that the expression levels of Mrp3 and/or Mrp4 were not altered in NAFLD or obese ZR rats compared to the controls [125, 129, 130].

In summary, the effects of NAFLD on Mrp2 expression were inconsistent or even conflicting. The discrepancy between Mrp2 mRNA and protein levels was also noted in the studies, indicating that post-transcriptional regulation plays an important role in regulating Mrp2 expression under the NAFLD condition. On the other hand, the expression of Mrp3 and Mrp4 was largely upregulated in NAFLD rodent models.

4.2.4 Oatps

Currently, there are seven studies evaluating the effects of NAFLD on the expression of Oatps. The expression levels of Oatp1a1 mRNA and/or protein were consistently decreased in six studies [117, 118, 125, 129, 132, 133], while one study showed no changes [126]. There are three studies investigating Oatp1a4. In one study, the expression levels of Oatp1a4 were significantly reduced at both mRNA and protein levels in *ob/ob* mice compared to lean control mice [118]. In another study, the expression levels of Oatp1a4 mRNA were increased but its protein levels were decreased in various mouse and rat NAFLD models compared to the corresponding control mice or rats [133]. On the other hand, no alterations in Oatp1a4 expression were detected in MCD-induced NAFLD rats [126]. The effects of NAFLD on the expression of Oatp1b2 were very much consistent among the five studies. Oatp1b2 expression was significantly downregulated in four studies [117, 126, 132, 133], while no alterations in Oatp1b2 expression were detected in one study [125]. There are three studies investigating Oatp2b1. One study with *ob/ob* mice reported that Oatp2b1 mRNA levels were significantly upregulated in *ob/ob* mice compared to the lean control mice [118]. However, other two studies showed that Oatp2b1 was downregulated in obese ZR rats compared to lean control rats [129, 132]. Taken together, Oatp1a1 and Oatp1b2 were consistently downregulated, while the effects on Oatp1a4 and Oatp2b1 were inconsistent in NAFLD rodents.

5. Alterations in bile acid regulators in subjects with NAFLD

Bile acid synthesis is tightly regulated by multiple signaling pathways, mainly the FXR/SHP [134, 135] and FGF19/FGFR4 [136, 137] negative feedback loops (**Figure 2**). In the liver, activation of FXR by bile acids induces SHP expression, which in turn represses CYP7A1 expression, leading to reduced bile acid synthesis. In the intestine, activation of FXR by bile acids upregulates FGF19 (FGF15 in rodents). After entering the circulation, FGF19 binds to FGFR4 in the liver to activate the downstream signaling, which subsequently inhibits CYP7A1 expression, resulting in decreased bile acid synthesis. Those two negative feedback regulatory loops play critical roles in regulating bile acid synthesis and maintaining bile acid homeostasis. Impairment or dysregulation of the FXR/SHP and FGF19/FGFR4 signaling pathways interrupts bile acid balance.

5.1 FXR/SHP signaling pathway

5.1.1 In human

Most of the human clinical studies revealed that the FXR/SHP signaling pathway was dysregulated in patients with NAFLD. In one study with 10 healthy controls, 39 steatotic, and 59 NASH patients, both FXR and SHP mRNA levels were significantly downregulated [94]. In two studies with 20 or 11 normal control subjects and 20 NAFLD or 16 NASH patients, the expression levels of FXR were significantly deceased in NAFLD or NASH patients compared to control subjects [101, 138]. However, the expression levels of SHP remain comparable between the control subjects and NAFLD or NASH patients, indicating that the FXR signaling is impaired in NAFLD or NASH patients [101, 138]. In a study with 33 children (19 NAFLD patients and 14 control children), the FXR protein levels were gradually decreased from control subjects to steatotic to NASH patients, indicating the worsening of FXR signaling as NAFLD progresses [139]. Consistently, in a study with 20 simple steatosis and 20 NASH patients, the FXR protein expression levels were significantly decreased in NASH patients compared to the patients with simple steatosis, although at the mRNA level, FXR expression was higher in patients with NASH than those in patients with simple steatosis [127]. On the other hand, in one study with 26 controls and 32 NASH patients, no differences were detected in the expression of both FXR and SHP between control and NASH subjects [91]. Finally, one study showed gender differences in FXR expression. A significant decrease in FXR expression was detected in female but not male NASH patients compared to control subjects, while SHP expression was significantly decreased in both male and female with NASH [122]. In summary, most of the studies revealed a decreased or impaired FXR signaling in patients with NAFLD, and such impairment gets worsening as NAFLD progresses from simple steatosis to NASH.

5.1.2 In rodent NAFLD models

Inconsistent results have been reported regarding the status of FXR signaling in NAFLD rodent models. In two studies with HFD or fructose-induced NAFLD mice, the FXR expression levels were significantly reduced in NAFLD mice compared to control mice [124, 140]. However, SHP expression remained unchanged in fructose-induced NAFLD mice while significantly increased in HFD-induced NAFLD mice. In another two studies with HFD/STZ or MCD-induced NAFLD rats, the FXR expression levels remained comparable between the NAFLD and control rats [125, 126]. Consistent with no changes in FXR expression, SHP expression was comparable between the two groups. In another study with *ob/ob* mice, FXR mRNA and protein were significantly increased in *ob/ob* mice compared to lean control mice, while no alterations in SHP expression was detected [118]. Finally, in a study with HFD-induced NAFLD mice, the FXR signaling status was investigated during the progression of NAFLD from simple steatosis to NASH, fibrosis, and hepatocellular carcinoma (HCC) on an HFD [141]. FXR signaling was strongly activated in the early stage of NAFLD (simple steatosis) evidenced by strong upregulation of FXR target genes including Bsep, Mrp2, and ATP-binding cassette subfamily G member 5 (Abcg5)/Abcg8. However, as NAFLD progressed, FXR signaling gradually decreased but was still higher than that in the control mice on regular diet. Taken together, the inconsistent results from the NAFLD rodent models indicate that the effects of NAFLD on the FXR signaling pathway are dependent on the methods by which NAFLD is induced as well as the species (mouse or rat).

5.2 FGF19/FGFR4 signaling pathway

A large number of clinical studies have demonstrated that the FGF19 signaling is dysregulated in patients with NAFLD. Serum FGF19 concentrations were significantly reduced in patients with simple steatosis or NASH compared to control subjects [88, 92, 101, 102, 139, 142–144]. The decreases in FGF19 concentrations were more severe in patients with NASH than the patients with steatosis, indicating the worsening of FGF19 signaling impairment as the NAFLD progresses from simple steatosis to NASH. On the other hand, there are two clinical studies showing that the fasting serum concentrations of FGF19 were not altered in patients with NAFLD compared to control subjects [107, 145]. Taken together, most of the clinical studies showed that the FGF19 signaling was reduced or impaired in patients with NAFLD.

6. Conclusions

A large body of evidence from clinical as well as preclinical studies has demonstrated that bile acid homeostasis is disrupted in subjects with NAFLD. The dysregulation of bile acids in patients with NAFLD gets worsening as the disease progresses from early stage simple steatosis to late stages NASH and NASH with fibrosis. Risk factors for NAFLD, especially obesity and insulin resistance, contribute to the dysregulation of bile acids in NAFLD patients.

Due to the complexity of bile acid regulation, small sample sizes in most of the clinical studies, variations in control subject selection, inherited differences in various rodent NAFLD models, and discrepancy in mRNA and protein levels of the target genes, inconsistent or even conflicting results, have been reported for serum and hepatic bile acid concentrations and compositions, as well as the expression levels of bile acid synthesis enzymes, transporters, and regulators. However, detailed examination and evaluation of the results from various studies, especially considering the characteristics of the studied subjects and the quality of each study, certain trends on alterations in serum and hepatic bile acid levels, bile acid synthesis, and regulation in patients with NAFLD are emerged.

As depicted in **Figure 3**, serum total bile acid concentrations are increased in patients with NAFLD, as a result of increased CYP7A1 expression and bile acid synthesis, elevated hepatic bile acids, and augment of MRP3 and MRP4 expression. Increased CYP7A1 expression and bile acid synthesis in patients with NAFLD are mainly due to the impairment of the FXR/SHP and FGF19/FGFR4 signaling pathways. Limited studies on investigating fecal and urine bile acids showed that both fecal and urine bile acid concentrations were elevated in patients with NAFLD, consistent with increased serum and hepatic bile acid levels in those patients.

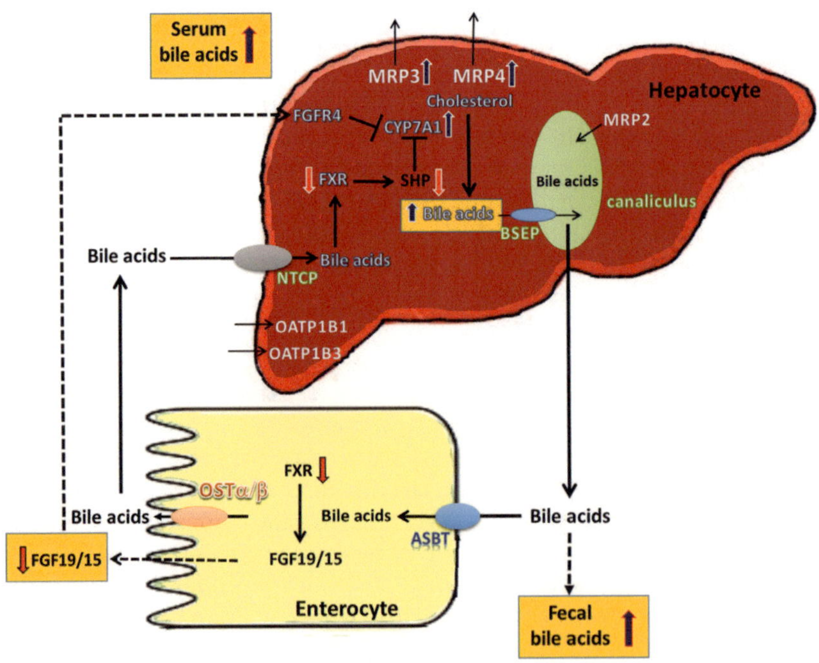

Figure 3.
Effects of NAFLD on serum, hepatic, and fecal bile acid concentrations as well as on bile acid synthesis (CYP7A1), transporters (MRP3 and MRP4), and regulators (FXR, SHP, FGF19/15).

7. Guidance for future studies

Future studies with high quality and large sample size are needed to solidify the trends depicted in **Figure 3**. The following points should be considered in the design of the future studies and interpretation of the findings. First, limited studies with children and adolescents revealed a different feature in bile acid dysregulation from adults with NAFLD. In contrast to the findings in adults, serum bile acid levels decrease in the early stage of NAFLD, followed by an increase as NAFLD progresses to fibrosis but the levels remain lower than those in the healthy control children. The effects of NAFLD on bile acid regulation appear different in children from adults. Second, the effects of NAFLD on bile acid homeostasis are stage dependent. No or mild effects of simple steatosis on bile acid regulation were detected, while significant alterations in bile acids are mostly detected in patients with NASH. A large percentage of previous studies did not separate the steatotic and NASH patients in the test groups, which certainly complicates the analysis and interpretation of data. Third, as risk factors for NAFLD, obesity and insulin resistance/diabetes are often associated with NAFLD. It is well documented that obesity and insulin resistance directly cause dysregulation of bile acids. Therefore, those risk factors should be adjusted or matched in the control group in order to reveal the exact effects of NAFLD on bile acid homeostasis. Among the clinical studies reported, only one study was conducted with a matched control group, in which a different conclusion was reached that NASH has no effects on bile acid regulation [93]. Fourth, in future studies using NAFLD rodent models, it should be emphasized that species differences between rodents and human and even between mouse and rat exist, especially in the effects of NAFLD on bile acid transporter expression. Finally, in the investigation of gene expression, both mRNA and protein levels should be detected and quantified for the target genes. Most of the previous studies only evaluated the mRNA levels. However, discrepancy between the mRNA and protein levels is often detected in studies investigating both levels. It appears that under the NAFLD condition, posttranscriptional regulation plays a predominant role in regulating the genes involved in bile acid synthesis, transport, and regulation.

Acknowledgements

This work was supported by the National Institutes of Health (NIH) Grants R01DK087755, R01CA213419 and R01GM061988.

Conflict of interest

The authors have no conflict of interest.

Author details

Xinmu Zhang and Ruitang Deng*
Department of Biomedical and Pharmaceutical Sciences, College of Pharmacy, University of Rhode Island, Kingston, RI, USA

*Address all correspondence to: dengr@uri.edu

IntechOpen

© 2018 The Author(s). Licensee IntechOpen. This chapter is distributed under the terms of the Creative Commons Attribution License (http://creativecommons.org/licenses/by/3.0), which permits unrestricted use, distribution, and reproduction in any medium, provided the original work is properly cited.

References

[1] Williams CD, Stengel J, Asike MI, Torres DM, Shaw J, Contreras M, et al. Prevalence of nonalcoholic fatty liver disease and nonalcoholic steatohepatitis among a largely middle-aged population utilizing ultrasound and liver biopsy: A prospective study. Gastroenterology. 2011;**140**:124-131. DOI: 10.1053/j.gastro.2010.09.038

[2] Younossi ZM, Koenig AB, Abdelatif D, Fazel Y, Henry L, Wymer M. Global epidemiology of nonalcoholic fatty liver disease-meta-analytic assessment of prevalence, incidence, and outcomes. Hepatology. 2016;**64**(1):73-84. DOI: 10.1002/hep.28431

[3] Schwimmer JB, Deutsch R, Kahen T, Lavine JE, Stanley C, Behling C. Prevalence of fatty liver in children and adolescents. Pediatrics. 2006;**118**:1388-1393. DOI: 10.1542/peds.2006-1212

[4] Temple JL, Cordero P, Li J, Nguyen V, Oben JA. A guide to non-alcoholic fatty liver disease in childhood and adolescence. International Journal of Molecular Sciences. 2016;**17**(6):947. DOI: 10.3390/ijms17060947

[5] Brunt EM, Janney CG, Di Bisceglie AM, Neuschwander-Tetri BA, Bacon BR. Nonalcoholic steatohepatitis: A proposal for grading and staging the histological lesions. American Journal of Gastroenterology. 1999;**94**:2467-2474. DOI: 10.1111/j.1572_0241.1999.01377.x

[6] Bellentani S. The epidemiology of non-alcoholic fatty liver disease. Liver International. 2017;**37**(S1):81-84. DOI: 10.1111/liv.13299

[7] Streba LA, Vere CC, Rogoveanu I, Streba CT. Nonalcoholic fatty liver disease, metabolic risk factors, and hepatocellular carcinoma: An open question. World Journal of Gastroenterology. 2015;**21**:4103-4110. DOI: 10.3748/wjg.v21.i14.4103

[8] Farrell GC. The liver and the waistline: Fifty years of growth. Journal of Gastroenterology and Hepatology. 2009;**24**:S105-S118. DOI: 10.1111/j.1440-1746.2009.06080.x

[9] Kim D, Chung GE, Kwak MS, Seo HB, Kang JH, Kim W, et al. Body fat distribution and risk of incident and regressed nonalcoholic fatty liver disease. Clinical Gastroenterology and Hepatology. 2016;**14**:132-138.e4. DOI: 10.1016/j.cgh.2015.07.024

[10] Yu SJ, Kim W, Kim D, Yoon JH, Lee K, Kim JH, et al. Visceral obesity predicts significant fibrosis in patients with nonalcoholic fatty liver disease. Medicine (Baltimore). 2015;**94**:e2159. DOI: 10.1097/MD.0000000000002159

[11] Hazlehurst JM, Woods C, Marjot T, Cobbold JF, Tomlinson JW. Non-alcoholic fatty liver disease and diabetes. Metabolism. 2016;**65**:1096-1108. DOI: 10.1016/j.metabol.2016.01.001

[12] Cusi K. Nonalcoholic fatty liver disease in type 2 diabetes mellitus. Current Opinion in Endocrinology, Diabetes and Obesity. 2009;**16**:141-149. DOI: 10.1097/MED.0b013e3283293015

[13] Portillo-Sanchez P, Bril F, Maximos M, Lomonaco R, Biernacki D, Orsak B, et al. High prevalence of nonalcoholic fatty liver disease in patients with type 2 diabetes mellitus and normal plasma aminotransferase levels. Bile acids: Natural ligands for an orphan. Nuclear Receptor. 2015;**100**:2231-2238. DOI: 10.1210/jc.2014-2739

[14] Parks DJ, Blanchard SG, Bledsoe RK, Chandra G, Consler TG, Kliewer SA, et al. Bile acids: Natural ligands for

an orphan nuclear receptor. Science. 1999;**284**:1365-1368. DOI: 10.1126/science.284.5418.1365

[15] Makishima M, Okamoto AY, Repa JJ, Tu H, Learned RM, Luk A, et al. Identification of a nuclear receptor for bile acids. Science. 1999;**284**:1362-1365. DOI: 10.1126/science.284.5418.1362

[16] Houten SM, Watanabe M, Auwerx J. Endocrine functions of bile acids. The EMBO Journal. 2006;**25**:1419-1425. DOI: 10.1038/sj.emboj.7601049

[17] Zhang Y, Edwards PA. FXR signaling in metabolic disease. FEBS Letters. 2008;**582**:10-18. DOI: 10.1016/j.febslet.2007.11.015

[18] Chiang JY. Bile acid metabolism and signaling. Comprehensive Physiology. 2013;**3**:1191-1212. DOI: 10.1002/cphy.c120023

[19] Chávez-Talavera O, Tailleux A, Lefebvre P, Staels B. Bile acid control of metabolism and inflammation in obesity, type 2 diabetes, dyslipidemia, and nonalcoholic fatty liver disease. Gastroenterology. 2017;**152**:1679-1694.e3. DOI: 10.1053/j.gastro.2017.01.055

[20] Schubert K, OldeDamink SWM, von Bergen M, Schaap FG. Interactions between bile salts, gut microbiota, and hepatic innate immunity. Immunological Reviews. 2017;**279**:23-35. DOI: 10.1111/imr.12579

[21] Vavassori P, Mencarelli A, Renga B, Distrutti E, Fiorucci S. The bile acid receptor FXR is a modulator of intestinal innate immunity. The Journal of Immunology. 2009;**183**:6251-6261. DOI: 10.4049/jimmunol.0803978

[22] Fiorucci S, Cipriani S, Mencarelli A, Renga B, Distrutti E, Baldelli F. Counter-regulatory role of bile acid activated receptors in immunity and inflammation. Current Molecular Medicine. 2010;**10**:579-595. DOI: 10.2174/1566524011009060579

[23] Li M, Cai SY, Boyer JL. Mechanisms of bile acid mediated inflammation in the liver. Molecular Aspects of Medicine. 2017;**56**:45-53. DOI: 10.1016/j.mam.2017.06.001

[24] Zhu C, Fuchs CD, Halilbasic E, Trauner M. Bile acids in regulation of inflammation and immunity: Friend or foe? Clinical and Experimental Rheumatology. 2016;**34**(4 Suppl 98):25-31

[25] Huang W, Ma K, Zhang J, Qatanani M, Cuvillier J, Liu J, et al. Nuclear receptor-dependent bile acid signaling is required for normal liver regeneration. Science. 2006;**312**:233-236. DOI: 10.1126/science.1121435

[26] Zhang L, Wang YD, Chen WD, Wang X, Lou G, Liu N, et al. Promotion of liver regeneration/repair by farnesoid X receptor in both liver and intestine in mice. Hepatology. 2012;**56**:2336-2343. DOI: 10.1002/hep.25905

[27] Fan M, Wang X, Xu G, Yan Q, Huang W. Bile acid signaling and liver regeneration. Biochimica et Biophysica Acta (BBA)—Gene Regulatory Mechanisms. 2015;**1849**:196-200. DOI: 10.1016/j.bbagrm.2014.05.021

[28] Chiang JY. Regulation of bile acid synthesis: Pathways, nuclear receptors, and mechanisms. Journal of Hepatology. 2004;**40**:539-551. DOI: 10.1016/j.jhep.2003.11.006

[29] Chiang JY. Recent advances in understanding bile acid homeostasis. F1000Research. 2017;**6**:2029. DOI: 10.12688/f1000research.12449.1. eCollection 2017

[30] Marin JJ, Macias RI, Briz O, Banales JM, Monte MJ. Bile acids in physiology, pathology and pharmacology. Current

Drug Metabolism. 2015;**17**:4-29. DOI: 10.2174/1389200216666151103115454

[31] Hofmann AF. The enterohepatic circulation of bile acids in mammals: Form and functions. Frontiers in Bioscience (Landmark Ed). 2009;**14**:2584-2598

[32] Dawson PA, Lan T, Rao A. Bile acid transporters. Journal of Lipid Research. 2009;**50**:2340-2357. DOI: 10.1194/jlr.R900012-JLR200

[33] Gonzalez FJ. Nuclear receptor control of enterohepatic circulation. Comprehensive Physiology. 2012;**2**: 2811-2828. DOI: 10.1002/cphy.c120007

[34] Halilbasic E, Claudel T, Trauner M. Bile acid transporters and regulatory nuclear receptors in the liver and beyond. Journal of Hepatology. 2013;**58**:155-168. DOI: 10.1016/j.jhep.2012.08.002

[35] Fuchs M. Bile acid regulation of hepatic physiology: III. Regulation of bile acid synthesis: Past progress and future challenges. American Journal of Physiology-Gastrointestinal and Liver Physiology. 2003;**284**:G551-G557. DOI: 10.1152/ajpgi.00468.2002

[36] Kullak-Ublick GA, Stieger B, Meier PJ. Enterohepatic bile salt transporters in normal physiology and liver disease. Gastroenterology. 2004;**126**(1):322-342. DOI: 10.1053/j.gastro.2003.06.005

[37] Douglas JG, Beckett GJ, Nimmo IA, Finlayson ND, Percy-Robb IW. Clinical value of bile salt tests in anicteric liver disease. Gut. 1981;**22**:141-148. DOI: 10.1136/gut.22.2.141

[38] Sugita T, Amano K, Nakano M, Masubuchi N, Sugihara M, Matsuura T. Analysis of the serum bile acid composition for differential diagnosis in patients with liver disease. Gastroenterology Research and Practice. 2015;**2015**:10. DOI: 10.1155/2015/717431

[39] Trottier J, Białek A, Caron P, Straka RJ, Heathcote J, Milkiewicz P, et al. Metabolomic profiling of 17 bile acids in serum from patients with primary biliary cirrhosis and primary sclerosing cholangitis: A pilot study. Digestive and Liver Disease. 2012;**44**:303-310. DOI: 10.1016/j.dld.2011.10.025

[40] Squires JE, Rudnick DA, Hardison RM, Horslen S, Ng VL, Alonso EM, et al. Glycodeoxycholic acid levels as prognostic biomarker in acetaminophen-induced acute liver failure patients. Toxicological Sciences. 2014;**142**: 436-444. DOI: 10.1093/toxsci/kfu195

[41] Bathena SP, Thakare R, Gautam N, Mukherjee S, Olivera M, Meza J, et al. Urinary bile acids as biomarkers for liver diseases I. Stability of the baseline profile in healthy subjects. Toxicological Sciences. 2015;**43**:296-307. DOI: 10.1093/toxsci/kfu227

[42] Schubert R, Schmidt KH. Structural changes in vesicle membranes and mixed micelles of various lipid compositions after binding of different bile salts. Biochemistry. 1988;**27**:8787-8794

[43] Sagawa H, Tazuma S, Kajiyama G. Protection against hydrophobic bile salt-induced cell membrane damage by liposomes and hydrophilic bile salts. American Journal of Physiology-Gastrointestinal and Liver Physiology. 1993;**264**:G835-G839. DOI: 10.1152/ajpgi.1993.264.5.G835

[44] Billington D, Evans CE, Godfrey PP, Coleman R. Effects of bile salts on the plasma membranes of isolated rat hepatocytes. Biochemical Journal. 1980;**188**:321-327

[45] Palmeira CM, Rolo AP. Mitochondrially-mediated toxicity of

bile acids. Toxicology. 2004;**203**:1-15. DOI: 10.1016/j.tox.2004.06.001

[46] Sokol RJ, Dahl R, Devereaux MW, Yerushalmi B, Kobak GE, Gumpricht E. Human hepatic mitochondria generate reactive oxygen species and undergo the permeability transition in response to hydrophobic bile acids. Journal of Pediatric Gastroenterology and Nutrition. 2005;**41**:235-243. DOI: 10.1097/01.MPG. 0000170600.80640.88

[47] Rolo AP, Palmeira CM, Wallace KB. Mitochondrially mediated synergistic cell killing by bile acids. Biochimica et Biophysica Acta (BBA)—Molecular Basis of Disease. 2003;**637**:127-132. DOI: 10.1016/S0925-4439(02)00224-7

[48] Sokol RJ, Winklhofer-Roob BM, Devereaux MW. Generation of hydroperoxides in isolated rat hepatocytes and hepatic mitochondria exposed to hydrophobic bile acids. Gastroenterology. 1995;**109**:1249-1256. DOI: 10.1016/0016-5085(95)90585-5

[49] Iizaka T, Tsuji M, Oyamada H, Morio Y, Oguchi K. Interaction between caspase-8 activation and endoplasmic reticulum stress in glycochenodeoxycholic acid-induced apoptotic HepG2 cells. Toxicology. 2007;**241**:146-156. DOI: 10.1016/j.tox.2007.08.095

[50] Adachi T, Kaminaga T, Yasuda H, Kamiya T, Hara H. The involvement of endoplasmic reticulum stress in bile acid-induced hepatocellular injury. Journal Clinical Biochemistry Nutrition. 2004;**54**:129-135. DOI: 10.3164/jcbn.13-46

[51] Tsuchiya S, Tsuji M, Morio Y, Oguchi K. Involvement of endoplasmic reticulum in glycochenodeoxycholic acid-induced apoptosis in rat hepatocytes. Toxicology Letters. 2006;**166**:140-169. DOI: 10.1016/j.toxlet.2006.06.006

[52] Gujral JS, Farhood A, Bajt ML. Neutrophils aggravate acute liver injury during obstructive cholestasis in bile duct-ligated mice. Hepatology. 2003;**38**:355-363. DOI: 10.1053/jhep.2003.50341

[53] Gujral JS, Liu J, Farhood A, Hinson JA, Jaeschke H. Functional importance of ICAM-1 in the mechanism of neutrophil-induced liver injury in bile duct-ligated mice. American Journal of Physiology-Gastrointestinal and Liver Physiology. 2004;**286**:G499-G507. DOI: 10.1152/ajpgi.00318.2003

[54] Allen K, Jaeschke H, Copple BL. Bile acids induce inflammatory genes in hepatocytes: A novel mechanism of inflammation during obstructive cholestasis. American Journal of Pathology. 2011;**178**:175-186. DOI: 10.1016/j.ajpath.2010.11.026

[55] Spivey JR, Bronk SF, Gores GJ. Glycochenodeoxycholate-induced lethal hepatocellular injury in rat hepatocytes. Role of ATP depletion and cytosolic free calcium. Journal of Clinical Investigation. 1993;**92**:17-24. DOI: 10.1172/JCI116546

[56] Yerushalmi B, Dahl R, Devereaux MW. Bile acid-induced rat hepatocyte apoptosis is inhibited by antioxidants and blockers of the mitochondrial permeability transition. Hepatology. 2001;**33**:616-626. DOI: 10.1053/jhep.2001.22702

[57] Rust C, Wild N, Bernt C, Vennegeerts T, Wimmer R, Beuers U. Bile acid-induced apoptosis in hepatocytes is caspase-6-dependent. The Journal of Biological Chemistry. 2009;**284**:2908-2916

[58] Perez MJ, Briz O. Bile-acid-induced cell injury and protection. World Journal Gastroenterology. 2009;**15**:1677-1689. DOI: 10.3748/wjg.15.1677

[59] Neale G, Lewis B, Weaver V, Panveliwalla D. Serum bile acids in liver disease. Gut. 1971;**12**(2):145-152. DOI: 10.1136/gut.12.2.145

[60] Orlando R, Azzalini L, Orando S, Lirussi F. Bile acids for non-alcoholic fatty liver disease and/or steatohepatitis. The Cochrane Database of Systematic Reviews. 2007;**1**:CD005160. DOI: 10.1002/14651858.CD005160.pub2

[61] Li Y, Jadhav K, Zhang Y. Bile acid receptors in non-alcoholic fatty liver disease. BiochemPharmacol. 2013;**86**:1517-1524. DOI: 10.1016/j.bcp.2013.08.015

[62] Zarrinpar A, Loomba R. Review article: The emerging interplay among the gastrointestinal tract, bile acids and incretins in the pathogenesis of diabetes and non-alcoholic fatty liver disease. Alimentary Pharmacology & Therapeutics. 2012;**36**:909-921. DOI: 10.1111/apt.12084

[63] Zhu Y, Liu H, Zhang M, Guo GL. Fatty liver diseases, bile acids, and FXR. Acta Pharmaceutica Sinica B. 2016;**6**:409-412. DOI: 10.1016/j.apsb.2016.07.008

[64] Yuan L, Bambha K. Bile acid receptors and nonalcoholic fatty liver disease. World Journal of Hepatology. 2015;**7**:2811-2818. DOI: 10.4254/wjh.v7.i28.2811

[65] Chow MD, Lee YH, Guo GL. The role of bile acids in nonalcoholic fatty liver disease and nonalcoholic steatohepatitis. Molecular Aspects of Medicine. 2017;**56**:34-44. DOI: 10.1016/j.mam.2017.04.004

[66] Arab JP, Karpen SJ, Dawson PA, Arrese M, Trauner M. Bile acids and nonalcoholic fatty liver disease: Molecular insights and therapeutic perspectives. Hepatology. 2017;**65**: 350-362. DOI: 10.1002/hep.28709

[67] Cruz-Ramón V, Chinchilla-López P, Ramírez-Pérez O, Méndez-Sánchez N. Bile acids in nonalcoholic fatty liver disease: New concepts and therapeutic advances. Annals of Hematology. 2017;**16**(Suppl. 1: s3-105):s58-s67. DOI: 10.5604/01.3001.0010.5498

[68] Molinaro A, Wahlström A, Marschall HU. Role of bile acids in metabolic control. Trends in Endocrinology & Metabolism. 2018;**29**:31-41. DOI: 10.1016/j.tem.2017.11.002

[69] Steinacher D, Claudel T, Trauner M. Therapeutic mechanisms of bile acids and nor-ursodeoxycholic acid in non-alcoholic fatty liver disease. Digestive Diseases. 2017;**35**:282-287. DOI: 10.1159/000454853

[70] Kim SG, Kim BK, Kim K, Fang S. Bile acid nuclear receptor farnesoid X receptor: Therapeutic target for nonalcoholic fatty liver disease. Endocrinology and Metabolism (Seoul). 2016;**31**:500-504. DOI: 10.3803/EnM.2016.31.4.500

[71] Perazzo H, Dufour JF. The therapeutic landscape of non-alcoholic steatohepatitis. Liver International. 2017;**37**:634-647. DOI: 10.1111/liv.13270

[72] Carr RM, Reid AE. FXR agonists as therapeutic agents for non-alcoholic fatty liver disease. Current Atherosclerosis Reports. 2015;**17**:500. DOI: 10.1007/s11883-015-0500-2

[73] Adorini L, Pruzanski M, Shapiro D. Farnesoid X receptor targeting to treat nonalcoholic steatohepatitis. Drug Discovery Today. 2012;**17**:988-997. DOI: 10.1016/j.drudis.2012.05.012

[74] Mudaliar S, Henry RR, Sanyal AJ, Morrow L, Marschall HU, Kipnes M, et al. Efficacy and safety of the farnesoid X receptor agonist obeticholic acid in patients with

type 2 diabetes and nonalcoholic fatty liver disease. Gastroenterology. 2013;**145**:574-582.e1. DOI: 10.1053/j.gastro.2013.05.042

[75] Neuschwander-Tetri BA, Loomba R, Sanyal AJ, Lavine JE, Van Natta ML, Abdelmalek MF, et al. Farnesoid X nuclear receptor ligand obeticholic acid for non-cirrhotic, non-alcoholic steatohepatitis (FLINT): A multicentre, randomised, placebo-controlled trial. Lancet. 2015;**385**:956-965. DOI: 10.1016/S0140-6736(14)61933-4

[76] Haedrich M, Dufour JF. UDCA for NASH: End of the story? Journal of Hepatology. 2011;**54**:856-858. DOI: 10.1016/j.jhep.2010.10.009

[77] Ratziu V. Treatment of NASH with ursodeoxycholic acid: Pro. Clinics and Research in Hepatology and Gastroenterology. 2012;**36**:S41-S45. DOI: 10.1016/S2210-7401(12)70020-7

[78] Leuschner UF, Lindenthal B, Herrmann G, Arnold JC, Rössle M, Cordes HJ, et al. High-dose ursodeoxycholic acid therapy for nonalcoholic steatohepatitis: A double-blind, randomized, placebo-controlled trial. Hepatology. 2010;**52**:472-479. DOI: 10.1002/hep.23727

[79] Adams LA, Angulo P, Petz J, Keach J, Lindor KD. A pilot trial of high-dose ursodeoxycholic acid in nonalcoholic steatohepatitis. Hepatology International. 2010;**4**:628-633. DOI: 10.1007/s12072-010-9195

[80] Russell DW, Setchell KDR. Bile acid biosynthesis. Biochemistry. 1992;**31**:4737-4749.

[81] Russell DW. The enzymes, regulation, and genetics of bile acid synthesis. Annual Review of Biochemistry. 2003;**72**:137-174. DOI: 10.1146/annurev.biochem.72.121801.161712

[82] Nakamura K. Bile acid transformation by anaerobic bacteria isolated from human feces and sewage by heat-treatment. lgakukenkyu. 1979;**49**:58-68

[83] Hirano S, Masuda N, Oda H, Imamura T. Transformation of bile acids by mixed microbial cultures from human feces and bile acid transforming activities of isolated bacteria strains. Microbiology Immunology. 1981;**25**:271-282. DOI: 10.1111/j.1348-0421.1981.tb00029.x

[84] Kole MM, Altosaar I. Conversion of chenodeoxycholic acid to ursodeoxycholic acid by Clostridium absonum in culture and by immobilized cells. FEMS. Microbiology Letters. 1985;**28**:69-72

[85] Xie G, Wang Y, Wang X, Zhao A, Chen T, Ni Y, et al. Profiling of serum bile acids in a healthy Chinese population using UPLC-MS/MS. Journal of Proteome Research. 2015;**14**:850-859. DOI: 10.1021/pr500920q

[86] Kalhan SC, Guo L, Edmison J, Dasarathy S, McCullough AJ, Hanson RW, et al. Plasma metabolomic profile in nonalcoholic fatty liver disease. Metabolism. 2011;**60**:404-413. DOI: 10.1016/j.metabol.2010.03.006

[87] Ferslew BC, Xie G, Johnston CK, Su M, Stewart PW, Jia W, et al. Altered bile acid metabolome in patients with nonalcoholic steatohepatitis. Digestive Diseases and Sciences. 2015;**60**: 3318-3328. DOI: 10.1007/s10620-015-3776-8

[88] Puri P, Daita K, Joyce A, Mirshahi F, Santhekadur PK, Cazanave S, et al. The presence and severity of nonalcoholic steatohepatitis is associated with specific changes in circulating bile acids. Hepatology. 2017. [Epub ahead of print]. DOI: 10.1002/hep.29359

[89] Ferslew BC, Johnston CK, Tsakalozou E, Bridges AS, Paine MF,

Jia W, et al. Altered morphine glucuronide and bile acid disposition in patients with nonalcoholic steatohepatitis. Clinical Pharmacology & Therapeutics. 2015;**97**:419-427. DOI: 10.1002/cpt.66

[90] Garcia-Canaveras JC, Donato MT, Castell JV, Lahoz A. Targeted profiling of circulating and hepatic bile acids in human, mouse, and rat using a UPLC-MRM-MS-validated method. Journal of Lipid Research. 2012;**53**:2231-2241. DOI: 10.1194/jlr.D028803

[91] Legry V, Francque S, Haas JT, Verrijken A, Caron S, Chávez-Talavera O, et al. Bile acid alterations are associated with insulin resistance, but not with NASH, in obese subjects. The Journal of Clinical Endocrinology and Metabolism. 2017;**102**:3783-3794. DOI: 10.1210/jc.2017-01397

[92] Friedrich D, Marschall HU, Lammert F. Response of fibroblast growth factor 19 and bile acid synthesis after a body weight-adjusted oral fat tolerance test in overweight and obese NAFLD patients: A non-randomized controlled pilot trial. BMC Gastroenterology. 2018;**18**:76. DOI: 10.1186/s12876-018-0805-z

[93] Dasarathy S, Yang Y, McCullough AJ, Marczewski S, Bennett C, Kalhan SC. Elevated hepatic fatty acid oxidation, high plasma fibroblast growth factor 21, and fasting bile acids in nonalcoholic steatohepatitis. European Journal of Gastroenterology & Hepatology. 2011;**23**:382-388. DOI: 10.1097/MEG.0b013e328345c8c7

[94] Bechmann LP, Kocabayoglu P, Sowa JP, Sydor S, Best J, Schlattjan M, et al. Free fatty acids repress small heterodimer partner (SHP) activation and adiponectin counteracts bile acid-induced liver injury in superobese patients with nonalcoholic steatohepatitis. Hepatology. 2013;**57**:1394-1406. DOI: 10.1002/hep.26225

[95] Vincent RP, Omar S, Ghozlan S, Taylor DR, Cross G, Sherwood RA, et al. Higher circulating bile acid concentrations in obese patients with type 2 diabetes. Annals of Clinical Biochemistry. 2013;**50**:360-364. DOI: 10.1177/0004563212473450

[96] Ma H, Patti ME. Bile acids, obesity, and the metabolic syndrome. Best Practice & Research in Clinical Gastroenterology. 2014;**28**:573-583. DOI: 10.1016/j.bpg.2014.07.004

[97] Zhang L, Li M, Zhan L, Lu X, Liang L, Su B, et al. Plasma metabolomic profiling of patients with diabetes-associated cognitive decline. PLoS One. 2015;**10**:e0126952. DOI: 10.1371/journal.pone.0126952

[98] Steiner C, Othman A, Saely CH, Rein P, Drexel H, von Eckardstein A, et al. Bile acid metabolites in serum: Intraindividual variation and associations with coronary heart disease, metabolic syndrome and diabetes mellitus. PLoS One. 2011;**6**:e25006. DOI: 10.1371/journal.pone.0025006

[99] Prawitt J, Caron S, Staels B. Bile acid metabolism and the pathogenesis of type 2 diabetes. Current Diabetes Reports. 2011;**11**:160-166. DOI: 10.1007/s11892-011-0187-x

[100] de Leon MP, Ferenderes R, Carulli N. Bile lipid composition and bile acid pool size in diabetes. American Journal of Digestive Diseases. 1978;**23**:710-716

[101] Jiao N, Baker SS, Chapa-Rodriguez A, Liu W, Nugent CA, Tsompana M, et al. Suppressed hepatic bile acid signalling despite elevated production of primary and secondary bile acids in NAFLD. Gut. 2017;67:1881-1891. DOI: 10.1136/gutjnl-2017-314307

[102] Jahnel J, Zöhrer E, Alisi A, Ferrari F, Ceccarelli S, De Vito R, et al. Serum bile acid levels in children with

nonalcoholic fatty liver disease. Journal of Pediatric Gastroenterology and Nutrition. 2015;**61**:85-90. DOI: 10.1097/MPG.0000000000000774

[103] Lu LP, Wan YP, Xun PC, Zhou KJ, Chen C, Cheng SY, et al. Serum bile acid level and fatty acid composition in Chinese children with non-alcoholic fatty liver disease. Journal of Digestive Diseases. 2017;**18**:461-471. DOI: 10.1111/1751-2980.12494

[104] Aranha MM, Cortez-Pinto H, Costa A, da Silva IB, Camilo ME, de Moura MC, et al. Bile acid levels are increased in the liver of patients with steatohepatitis. European Journal of Gastroenterology & Hepatology. 2008;**20**:519-525. DOI: 10.1097/MEG.0b013e3282f4710a

[105] Lake AD, Novak P, Shipkova P, Aranibar N, Robertson D, Reily MD, et al. Decreased hepatotoxic bile acid composition and altered synthesis in progressive human nonalcoholic fatty liver disease. Toxicology and Applied Pharmacology. 2013;**268**: 132-140. DOI: 10.1016/j.taap.2013.01.022

[106] Valanejad L, Ghareeb M, Shiffka S, Nadolny C, Chen Y, Guo L, et al. Dysregulation of Δ4-3-oxosteroid 5β-reductase in diabetic patients: Implications and mechanisms. Molecular and Cellular Endocrinology. 2018;**470**:127-141. DOI: 10.1016/j.mce.2017.10.005

[107] Mouzaki M, Wang AY, Bandsma R, Comelli EM, Arendt BM, Zhang L, et al. Bile acids and dysbiosis in non-alcoholic fatty liver disease. PLoS One. 2016;**11**:e0151829. DOI: 10.1371/journal.pone.0151829. eCollection 2016

[108] Han S, Zhang R, Jain R, Shi H, Zhang L, Zhou G, et al. Circadian control of bile acid synthesis by a KLF15-Fgf15 axis. Nature Communications. 2015;**6**:7231. DOI: 10.1038/ncomms8231

[109] Setchell KD, Lawson AM, Blackstock EJ, Murphy GM. Diurnal changes in serum unconjugated bile acids in normal man. Gut. 1982;**23**:637-642

[110] Gälman C, Angelin B, Rudling M. Bile acid synthesis in humans has a rapid diurnal variation that is asynchronous with cholesterol synthesis. Gastroenterology. 2005;**129**:1445-1453

[111] Noshiro M, Nishimoto M, Okuda K. Rat liver cholesterol 7 alpha-hydroxylase. Pretranslational regulation for circadian rhythm. Journal Biology Chemistry. 1990;**265**:10036-10041

[112] Ferrell JM, Chiang JY. Short-term circadian disruption impairs bile acid and lipid homeostasis in mice. Cell Molecular Gastroenterol Hepatology. 2015;**1**:664-677. DOI: 10.1016/j.jcmgh.2015.08.003

[113] Santhekadur PK, Kumar DP, Sanyal AJ. Preclinical models of non-alcoholic fatty liver disease. The Journal of Hepatology. 2018;**68**:230-237. DOI: 10.1016/j.jhep.2017.10.031

[114] Van Herck MA, Vonghia L, Francque SM. Animal models of nonalcoholic fatty liver disease-a starter's guide. Nutrients. 2017;**9**(10). pii: E1072. DOI: 10.3390/nu9101072

[115] Rasselli E, Canesi L, Portincasa P, Voci A, Vergani L, Demori I. Models of non-alcoholic fatty liver disease and potential translational value: The effects of 3,5-L-diiodothyronine. Annals of Hepatology. 2017;**16**:707-719. DOI: 10.5604/01.3001.0010.2713

[116] Jia X, Suzuki Y, Naito H, Yetti H, Kitamori K, Hayashi Y, et al. A possible role of chenodeoxycholic acid and glycine-conjugated bile acids in fibrotic

steatohepatitis in a dietary rat model. Digestive Diseases and Sciences. 2014;**59**:1490-1501. DOI: 10.1007/s10620-014-3028-3

[117] Tanaka N, Matsubara T, Krausz KW, Patterson AD, Gonzalez FJ. Disruption of phospholipid and bile acid homeostasis in mice with nonalcoholic steatohepatitis. Hepatology. 2012;**56**:118-129. DOI: 10.1002/hep.25630

[118] Martin IV, Schmitt J, Minkenberg A, Mertens JC, Stieger B, Mullhaupt B, et al. Bile acid retention and activation of endogenous hepatic farnesoid-X-receptor in the pathogenesis of fatty liver disease in ob/ob-mice. Journal of Biological Chemistry. 2010;**391**: 1441-1449. DOI: 10.1515/BC.2010.141

[119] Rasineni K, Penrice DD, Natarajan SK, McNiven MA, McVicker BL, Kharbanda KK, et al. Alcoholic vs non-alcoholic fatty liver in rats: Distinct differences in endocytosis and vesicle trafficking despite similar pathology. BMC Gastroenterology. 2016;**16**:27. DOI: 10.1186/s12876-016-0433-4

[120] Wruck W, Adjaye J. Meta-analysis reveals up-regulation of cholesterol processes in non-alcoholic and down-regulation in alcoholic fatty liver disease. World Journal of Gastroenterology. 2017;**9**:443-454. DOI: 10.4254/wjh.v9.i8.443

[121] Min HK, Kapoor A, Fuchs M, Mirshahi F, Zhou H, Maher J, et al. Increased hepatic synthesis and dysregulation of cholesterol metabolism is associated with the severity of nonalcoholic fatty liver disease. Cell Metabolism. 2012;**15**:665-674. DOI: 10.1016/j.cmet.2012.04.004

[122] Okushin K, Tsutsumi T, Enooku K, Fujinaga H, Kado A, Shibahara J, et al. The intrahepatic expression levels of bile acid transporters are inversely correlated with the histological progression of nonalcoholic fatty liver disease. Journal of Gastroenterology. 2016;**51**:808-818. DOI: 10.1007/s00535-015-1148-y

[123] Axelson M, Bjorkhem I, Reihner E, Einarsson K. The plasma level of 7 alpha-hydroxy-4-cholesten-3-one reflects the activity of hepatic cholesterol 7 alpha-hydroxylase in man. FEBS Letters. 1991;**284**:216-218. DOI: 10.1016/0014-5793(91)80688-Y

[124] Wang C, Tao Q, Wang X, Wang X, Zhang X. Impact of high-fat diet on liver genes expression profiles in mice model of nonalcoholic fatty liver disease. Environmental Toxicology and Pharmacology. 2016;**45**:52-62. DOI: 10.1016/j.etap.2016.05.014

[125] Pozzo L, Vornoli A, Coppola I, Croce CM, Giorgetti L, Gervasi PG, et al. Effect of HFD/STZ on expression of genes involved in lipid, cholesterol and glucose metabolism in rats. Life Sciences. 2016;**166**:149-156. DOI: 10.1016/j.lfs.2016.09.022

[126] Lionarons DA, Heger M, van Golen RF, Alles LK, van der Mark VA, Kloek JJ, et al. Simple steatosis sensitizes cholestatic rats to liver injury and dysregulates bile salt synthesis and transport. Scientific Reports. 2016;**6**:31829. DOI: 10.1038/srep31829

[127] Aguilar-Olivos NE, Carrillo-Córdova D, Oria-Hernández J, Sánchez-Valle V, Ponciano-Rodríguez G, Ramírez-Jaramillo M, et al. The nuclear receptor FXR, but not LXR, up-regulates bile acid transporter expression in non-alcoholic fatty liver disease. Annals of Hepatology. 2015;**14**:487-493

[128] Sookoian S, Castaño G, Gianotti TF, Gemma C, Pirola CJ. Polymorphisms of MRP2 (ABCC2) are associated with susceptibility to nonalcoholic fatty liver disease. Journal of Nutritional Biochemistry. 2009;**20**:765-770. DOI: 10.1016/j.jnutbio.2008.07.005

[129] Geier A, Dietrich CG, Grote T, Beuers U, Prüfer T, Fraunberger P, et al. Characterization of organic anion transporter regulation, glutathione metabolism and bile formation in the obese Zucker rat. Journal of Hepatology. 2005;**43**:1021-1130. DOI: 10.1016/j.jhep.2005.05.031

[130] Pizarro M, Balasubramaniyan N, Solís N, Solar A, Duarte I, Miquel JF, et al. Bile secretory function in the obese Zucker rat: Evidence of cholestasis and altered canalicular transport function. Gut. 2004;**53**:1837-1843. DOI: 10.1136/gut.2003.037689

[131] Figge A, Lammert F, Paigen B, Henkel A, Matern S, Korstanje R, et al. Hepatic overexpression of murine Abcb11 increases hepatobiliary lipid secretion and reduces hepatic steatosis. Journal of Biological Chemistry. 2004;**279**:2790-2799. DOI: 10.1074/jbc.M307363200

[132] Fisher CD, Lickteig AJ, Augustine LM, Oude Elferink RP, Besselsen DG, Erickson RP, et al. Experimental non-alcoholic fatty liver disease results in decreased hepatic uptake transporter expression and function in rats. European Journal of Pharmacology. 2009;**613**:119-127. DOI: 10.1016/j.ejphar.2009.04.002

[133] Canet MJ, Hardwick RN, Lake AD, Dzierlenga AL, Clarke JD, Cherrington NJ. Modeling human nonalcoholic steatohepatitis-associated changes in drug transporter expression using experimental rodent models. Drug Metabolism and Disposition. 2014;**42**:586-695. DOI: 10.1124/dmd.113.055996

[134] Goodwin B, Jones SA, Price RR, Watson MA, McKee DD, Moore LB, et al. A regulatory cascade of the nuclear receptors FXR, SHP-1, and LRH-1 represses bile acid biosynthesis. Molecular Cell. 2000;**6**:517-526

[135] Lu TT, Makishima M, Repa JJ, Schoonjans K, Kerr TA, Auwerx J, et al. Molecular basis for feedback regulation of bile acid synthesis by nuclear receptors. Molecular Cell. 2000;**6**:507-515

[136] Holt JA, Luo G, Billin AN, Bisi J, McNeill YY, Kozarsky KF, et al. Definition of a novel growth factor-dependent signal cascade for the suppression of bile acid biosynthesis. Genes & Development. 2003;**17**:1581-1591

[137] Song KH, Li T, Owsley E, Strom S, Chiang JY. Bile acids activate fibroblast growth factor 19 signaling in human hepatocytes to inhibit cholesterol 7alpha-hydroxylase gene expression. Hepatology. 2009;**49**:297-305. DOI: 10.1002/hep.22627

[138] Yang ZX, Shen W, Sun H. Effects of nuclear receptor FXR on the regulation of liver lipid metabolism in patients with non-alcoholic fatty liver disease. Hepatology International. 2010;**4**:741-748. DOI: 10.1007/s12072-010-9202-6

[139] Nobili V, Alisi A, Mosca A, Della Corte C, Veraldi S, De Vito R, et al. Hepatic farnesoid X receptor protein level and circulating fibroblast growth factor 19 concentration in children with NAFLD. International Journal. 2018;**38**:342-349. DOI: 10.1111/liv.13531

[140] Volynets V, Spruss A, Kanuri G, Wagnerberger S, Bischoff SC, Bergheim I. Protective effect of bile acids on the onset of fructose-induced hepatic steatosis in mice. Journal of Lipid Research. 2010;**51**:3414-3424. DOI: 10.1194/jlr.M007179

[141] Cazanave S, Podtelezhnikov A, Jensen K, Seneshaw M, Kumar DP, Min HK, et al. The transcriptomic signature of disease development and progression of nonalcoholic fatty liver disease.

Scientific Reports. 2017;7:17193. DOI: 10.1038/s41598-017-17370-6

[142] Alisi A, Ceccarelli S, Panera N, Prono F, Petrini S, De Stefanis C, et al. Association between serum atypical fibroblast growth factors 21 and 19 and pediatric nonalcoholic fatty liver disease. PLoS One. 2013;**8**:e67160. DOI: 10.1371/journal.pone.0067160. Print 2013

[143] Eren F, Kurt R, Ermis F, Atug O, Imeryuz N, Yilmaz Y. Preliminary evidence of a reduced serum level of fibroblast growth factor 19 in patients with biopsy-proven nonalcoholic fatty liver disease. Clinical Biochemistry. 2012;**45**:655-658. DOI: 10.1016/j.clinbiochem.2012.03.019

[144] Wojcik M, Janus D, Dolezal-Oltarzewska K, Kalicka-Kasperczyk A, Poplawska K, Drozdz D, et al. A decrease in fasting FGF19 levels is associated with the development of non-alcoholic fatty liver disease in obese adolescents. Journal of Pediatric Endocrinology and Metabolism. 2012;**25**:1089-1093. DOI: 10.1515/jpem-2012-0253

[145] Schreuder TC, Marsman HA, Lenicek M, van Werven JR, Nederveen AJ, Jansen PL, et al. The hepatic response to FGF19 is impaired in patients with nonalcoholic fatty liver disease and insulin resistance. American Journal of Physiology—Gastrointestinal and Liver Physiology. 2010;**298**:G440-G445. DOI: 10.1152/ajpgi.00322.2009

Chapter 5

The Rise in the Prevalence of Nonalcoholic Fatty Liver Disease and Hepatocellular Carcinoma

Zaki A. Sherif

Abstract

Nonalcoholic fatty liver disease (NAFLD) affects a third of the world's population and its rapid rise parallels the increase in hepatocellular carcinoma (HCC). NAFLD replacing hepatitis C virus (HCV) infection as a leading indicator for liver transplantation (LT) in the United States. NAFLD is a spectrum of disease ranging from simple steatosis (NAFL) to nonalcoholic steatohepatitis (NASH), which can progress to advanced fibrosis (AF) and cirrhosis, culminating in HCC. The main clinical concern of public health administrators is that many patients who are unaware of NAFLD remain undiagnosed and risk developing end-stage liver disease (ESLD). Clinicians overly rely on surrogate liver enzymes to identify patients with NAFLD, allowing for substantial liver disease to go unnoticed and untreated. Furthermore, according to epidemiological studies, in patients diagnosed with NAFLD, ethnicity plays a role in complications and treatment response, and ethnic correlations with NAFLD are thoroughly underreported. Although liver biopsy is the gold standard method for appropriately diagnosing and staging NAFLD, most patients can be effectively diagnosed non-invasively with imaging modalities and integrated tests that are routinely available in the clinic today. This chapter discusses the current global rise in the rates of NAFLD and HCC; the current key findings incidences and the recommended diagnostic approaches and in therapeutic methods.

Keywords: obesity, cirrhosis, hepatocellular carcinoma (HCC), insulin resistance (IR), liver transplantation (LT), metabolic syndrome (MetS), nonalcoholic fatty liver disease (NAFLD), nonalcoholic steatohepatitis (NASH)

1. Introduction

The liver is a 1.5 kg reddish-brown biochemical processing plant of immense responsibilities that include protein synthesis, xenobiotic or drug metabolism, blood detoxification, and the release of bile acids for digestion. In short, the liver plays a key role in the hemostasis of the body by regulating the levels of sugar, protein, and fat that circulate in the blood. However, obesity, which must be carefully defined according to ethnic-specific BMI cut-off points, may alter normal liver physiology and lead to liver disease [1]. Obesity is at the intersection of the chronic liver disease pathway that includes diabetes, metabolic syndrome (MetS), nonalcoholic fatty liver disease (NAFLD), and hepatocellular carcinoma (HCC). The complex association between obesity and liver function involving NAFLD, HCC, histopathology, and genetic factors is the subject of several collaborative research investigations [2–7].

Over the past few decades, dramatic changes in lifestyle behaviors and health priorities have contributed to a significant rise in noncommunicable diseases such as obesity and NAFLD. Obesity is highly prevalent in the United States of America, estimated to represent between 30 and 38% of adults with a body mass index (BMI) greater than 30 kg/m^2 [8, 9]. Obesity is also a risk factor for metabolic syndrome (MetS), which increases hepatic triglyceride (TGs) depositions. NAFLD is the most common cause of impaired liver function in Western countries, affecting over one quarter of the population [10, 11]. Obesity is driving the rise of NAFLD and nonalcoholic steatohepatitis (NASH), the culmination of the fatty liver disease spectrum that is manifested by ballooning, scarring, cirrhosis, and finally liver failure and HCC [12]. It is estimated that globally the prevalence of NAFLD in the general population is 24–30% [13, 14]. Accounting for errors in accuracy that may exist in indirect measurement methodologies, in the United States, the prevalence of NAFLD in adults has risen from 18% in 1988–1991, to 29% in 1999–2000, to 31% in 2011–2012 [15]. However, the prevalence of NAFLD in the United States diagnosed by ultrasonography alone was estimated to be 24.13% (95% CI 19.73–29.15%) [16].

1.1 NAFLD definition

Nonalcoholic fatty liver disease (NAFLD) is a broad-spectrum disease ranging from fat infiltration of hepatocytes with no symptoms (simple steatosis aka nonalcoholic fatty liver, NAFL) to excess intrahepatic macroglobular and macrovesicular fat accumulation (5–10% by weight of liver) with aggravated inflammation (steatohepatitis aka nonalcoholic steatohepatitis, NASH) in the presence of little ethanol (typically <30 g per day for men and <20 g per day for women) or no alcohol consumption in the last 12 months [12, 17]. It should be noted, however, there is now convincing evidence demonstrating that even "safe" levels of alcohol consumption are associated with adverse health outcomes [17–20] suggesting that future studies should include only nondrinker individuals in the "NAFLD definition" [21]. Therefore, for NAFLD classification, the patient must show evidence of hepatic fat accumulation in the absence of declared chronic alcohol consumption, or drug use that can induce steatosis, or hereditary disorders. This NAFLD designation excludes both macrovesicular and microvesicular steatosis encompassing certain drugs, toxins, viral hepatitis B (HBV), hepatitis C (HCV) or human immunodeficiency virus (HIV) infections, celiac disease, α-1 antitrypsin deficiency, hepatobiliary infectious diseases, hepatolenticular degeneration, hepatic malignancies, genetic hemochromatosis, Wilson's disease, lipodystrophy, abetalipoproteinemia, Reye's syndrome, HELLP syndrome, or decompensated cirrhosis, which may contribute to secondary causes of steatosis and elevated liver enzymes [22–24]. Additional medications targeted for exclusion are estrogen, sodium valproate, nonsteroidal anti-inflammatory drugs (NSAIDs), calcium antagonists, perhexiline-maleate, and antiretroviral drugs [25–27]. Appropriate medical history must also be taken to exclude the uncommon causes of fatty liver secondary to treatment with drugs such as amiodarone, diltiazem, steroids, synthetic estrogens, tamoxifen, and highly active antiretroviral therapy; refeeding syndrome and total parenteral nutrition; severe weight loss after jejunoileal or gastric bypass; lipodystrophy; and other rare disorders [28]. There are also strong opinions for the exclusion of "whole-body system diseases" such as inflammatory bowel syndrome, hypothyroidism, and lipoatrophy [25] from the "secondary fatty liver diseases" category because they may also induce liver steatosis.

NAFLD can be distinguished from alcoholic steatohepatitis (ASH) by the absence of alcohol consumption and on histological markers such as sclerosing hyaline necrosis, hepatocyte ballooning, portal granulocytic inflammation, lobular inflammation, satellitosis, perisinusoidal fibrosis, Mallory-Denk bodies, and acute cholestasis among others [29–31]. However, it is important to note that NAFLD can also coexist with other liver diseases including HCV, hemochromatosis, and alcoholic liver disease, which can accelerate progression to end-stage liver disease (ESLD) [32].

1.2 The natural history of NAFLD

The pathophysiology of NAFLD and its variants is still incompletely understood thereby limiting the availability of effective diagnostic and therapeutic intervention. The ongoing persistence of obesity and the accompanying high rates of diabetes will increase the prevalence of NAFLD [33]. In many cases, the natural cause of the disease is the development of cirrhosis and ESLD as the population ages. Increased mortality rates have been reported in studies that compared NAFLD patients with a normal reference population [34–36]. The primary cause of death for NAFLD patients is cardiovascular disease followed by nonliver cancer, whereas the third leading cause of mortality is liver-related complications including cirrhosis [33]. The exact prevalence of fatty liver condition is not known, but population studies from the United States and China estimate that 28–30% of the general population has simple steatosis that carries a relatively benign prognosis and is measured using magnetic resonance spectroscopy (the most accurate imaging modality) and that 8% of the population has elevated alanine transaminase (ALT) [37, 38]. A follow-up of population-based studies examining the natural history of NAFLD patients in Minnesota revealed that 3.1% of the patients developed cirrhosis-related complications including ascites (2%), jaundice (2%), encephalopathy (2%), variceal bleeding (1%), and HCC (0.5%) [34]. Approximately 10–30% of those with steatosis develop NASH, and the development of NASH cirrhosis is associated with a poor long-term prognosis for 2.6% of them who will be at a risk of developing HCC [39–41]. Ten years following diagnosis, 45% will decompensate and the mortality rate for subjects with Child-Pugh A disease will be 20% [42]. Furthermore, besides having an increased liver-related mortality rate compared to the general population, patients with NASH also have an increased risk of cardiovascular death (15.5 vs. 7.5%, $p = 0.04$) [35]. Generally, NAFLD is a slowly progressing disease, which does not culminate in ESLD in most patients. Identifying those who will develop a complete liver failure is a difficult proposition [43]. NAFLD data are limited on predictors of clinical progression to NASH and beyond. Due to the compounding effect of obesity, prospective longitudinal studies are needed to help in the prediction of outcomes for individual patients. On the other hand, patients with NASH have a worse prognosis and attempts should be made to include them in clinical trials of novel treatments for this condition. The sequence of steps in liver disease commencing with steatosis and eventually culminating in HCC (i.e., ESLD) is presented in **Figure 1** [44].

1.3 NAFLD diagnosis and staging

The general classification of NAFLD as stated above and accepted by the American Association for the Study of Liver Diseases (AASLD) is a hepatic fat accumulation exceeding 5–10% by weight of the liver [45]. Accordingly, NAFLD diagnosis in the liver is based on: (i) the presence of simple steatosis, as determined by histological or imaging procedure; (ii) a total weekly consumption of less than 140 g of ethanol for men and less than 70 g for women in the last 12 months; and (iii) the absence of competing etiologies for simple liver steatosis and the absence of coexisting causes for chronic liver disease [46]. An appropriate diagnosis of

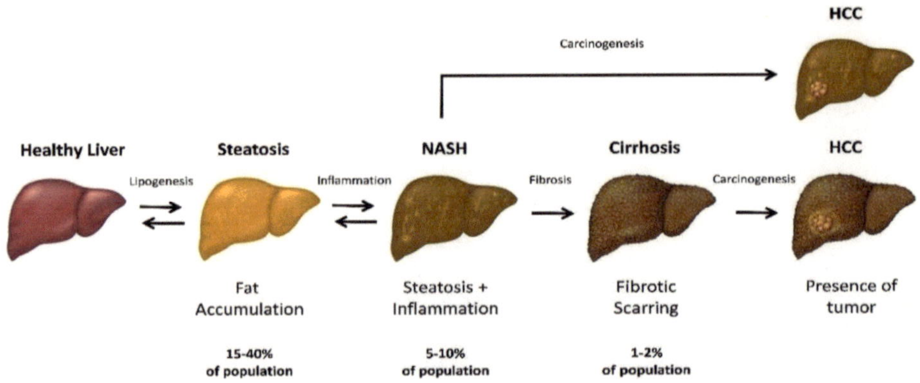

Figure 1.
The progression and stages of NAFLD (adapted from Baranova et al., [44]). Steatosis is the initial NAFLD stage and is characterized by excessive accumulation of fat in hepatocytes. Subsequent inflammatory conditions accelerate the progression to NASH followed by liver cirrhosis, which may lead to HCC. Both steatosis and NASH can reverse to NAFLD.

NAFLD, which is multifaceted, requires that there is evidence of hepatic steatosis upon imaging and histology or both and that other causes of liver disease including steatosis have been excluded [23].

The increasing prevalence of obesity in the past few decades has led to a surge in NAFLD, which manifests liver cells as bloated with droplets of fat. It has been reported that 70% of centrally obese patients with diabetes and hypertension (HTN) harbor steatohepatitis on liver biopsy [47]. Imaging has enabled the observation of central obesity in 70–80% of these subjects and in 50–80% of patients with type 2 diabetes mellitus (T2DM). NAFLD is typically asymptomatic; therefore, diagnosis usually follows the subsidiary finding of abnormal liver enzymes or steatosis on imaging. Early diagnosis of NAFLD requires skilled and informed practitioners to halt fibrosis progression to more advanced stages. Liver needle puncture biopsy, although invasive, is the gold standard. Less-invasive methods of image detection tools may not provide consistent information due to the subjective interpretations of the data by radiologists [48]. But imaging tools such as abdominal ultrasound (US), computed tomography (CT), and magnetic resonance imaging (MRI) are beginning to meet this need. Ultrasound or sonography is very effective in diagnosing steatosis where greater than 33% of hepatocytes are steatotic but can be unreliable with lesser degrees of steatosis [49]. The other imaging modalities such as CT or MRI can also detect hepatic steatosis even though they are not used in the evaluation of steatosis. Currently, the combination of MRI and proton magnetic resonance spectroscopy (MRI/^{1}H-MRS) is the most accurate noninvasive measuring tool of steatosis [50, 51]. ^{1}H-MRS, which defines NAFLD as hepatic fat accumulation (steatosis) >5% of total weight of the liver, is the most reliable quantitative tool. However, due to its prohibitive cost, it is not widely available. Ultrasonography, on the other hand, is the instrument of choice for most of the clinics due to its low cost and wide availability even though it is still relatively limited in the detection of inflammation, a more important and higher risk concern than steatosis for fibrosis, cirrhosis, and HCC [52, 53].

Controlled attenuation parameter (CAP), which is a novel ultrasound-based technique that assesses liver stiffness and steatosis simultaneously by employing transient elastography (TE) [54]. This CAP technique has been shown to accurately detect steatosis although its diagnostic threshold has not yet been determined. Obesity and diabetes are the main risk factors for NAFLD [55]. It has been reported that the presence of T2DM significantly increases the prevalence of NAFLD regardless of the diagnostic tool [56]. For example, using controlled attenuation parameter (CAP), the prevalence of NAFLD is estimated at 75% in T2DM population and 40% in the general population, whereas it is 65% and about 37% respectively when measured by ^{1}H-MRS. The prevalence rate goes down when assessed by liver ultrasound, computed tomography, and plasma ALT in that order [56].

In contrast, most global population studies base their NAFLD characterization on less sensitive and less specific surrogate markers of the disease including elevated liver-associated enzymes such as aspartate aminotransferase (AST) and alanine aminotransferase (ALT >40 IU/L in males; >31 IU/L in females) [57, 58]. Furthermore, serum ALT levels are within the range currently considered "normal" in a sizeable proportion of NAFLD subjects [59]. Typically, depending on the reference values from different laboratories, the broad range for normal AST is reported between 10 and 40 IU/L and ALT between 7 and 56 IU/L. This is because ALT usually falls (and AST may rise) as fibrosis progresses to cirrhosis. Mild elevations, which are generally asymptomatic, are considered to be 2–3 times higher than the normal range, and drastic elevations are 5 times higher than the upper limit of normal, which varies according to gender [60]. Moreover, the very selective measurement of ALT level based on race or ethnicity underscores the lack of effective surrogate markers for NAFLD/NASH in the absence of biopsy [61]. Therefore, an innovative approach is needed to use metabolic risk factors to identify subjects with NAFLD/NASH rather than relying on liver enzyme abnormalities.

There is an active research that is underway to discover serum biomarkers for NASH since it is associated with increased apoptosis and therefore blood markers of apoptosis may be instrumental in distinguishing NASH from simple steatosis [62]. Apoptosis activates caspases that cleave various substrates such as cytokeratin-18 (CK-18), a key intermediate filament protein in hepatocytes, that can be detected with an ELISA test using an M30 antibody to identify patients with NASH [63, 64]. However, liver biopsy provides a superior assessment of hepatic steatosis, hepatocellular injury, inflammation, and fibrosis as well as its ability to demonstrate the presence of hepatocyte ballooning and degeneration in association with steatosis as the key histological feature that distinguishes NASH from simple steatosis. Notwithstanding its limitations such as inherent variability in histologic assessment of NAFLD stage and activity, its invasiveness, its high possibility of complications related to liver damage, its proneness to sampling error generated by the operators, and its limitations in accessibility and reproducibility, liver biopsy is still the standard criterion for the most accurate diagnosis of NAFLD and NASH. Also, because only 7–30% of NAFLD patients in the world population had an indication of biopsy for accurate measurement, Younosis et al., re-evaluated and reported the global prevalence of NASH to be between 1.5 and 6.45% and the North American rate at an average of 8.69% (between 7.2 and 14.63%) [4, 65]. Regarding obesity, reports show that NASH can be verified by histological examination in about 47% of all NAFLD cases among obese individuals [66].

Liver fibrosis is the inordinate accretion of extracellular matrix proteins that include collagen in most types of liver disease including NAFLD. Fibrosis stage is a crucial histological variable to predict mortality. There are well-known independent predictors of fibrosis, which is a subway to chronic liver disease state. Some of these risk factors are age (>45–50), BMI (>28–30 kg/m^{2}), insulin resistance (IR), diabetes, and HTN [67]. Staging hepatic fibrosis is essential in all patients with NAFLD to identify individuals with advanced fibrosis (AF) who may later develop liver-related complications such as hepatocellular dysfunction and portal hypertension

(PHTN). A noninvasive and an indirect assessment, which is performed in all liver disease patients including children, may include blood tests such as liver function tests (low albumin), complete blood count (thrombocytopenia and neutropenia), and coagulation profile (prolonged prothrombin time) [68]. Among the diagnostic tools used to measure the prevalence of AF in the setting of T2DM versus the general population, vibration-controlled transient elastography shows the highest prevalence rate followed by NAFLD fibrosis score and FibroTest in that order. It should be noted that the prevalence of T2DM significantly increases the prevalence of AF in similar ways to NAFLD [56].

The most widespread clinically implemented histological grading and staging system is the 'NAFLD activity score' (NAS) [6] (see **Table 1**). More recently, the SAF score encompassing an assessment of steatosis (S), activity (A), and fibrosis (F) has been used to produce more accurate measurements of NASH [5]. These recent developments underscore the fact that NAFLD patients can be diagnosed and staged effectively using noninvasive strategies even though liver biopsy can still be applied for individuals with dubious diagnostic tests or if noninvasive staging is unspecified [69]. However, there is no widely available simple blood test or imaging modality that can differentiate simple steatosis from NASH.

In summary, early diagnosis of NAFLD is essential to halting the progression of the disease. Biopsy is intrusive and therefore cannot be routinely applied. Ultrasound (sonography) and magnetic resonance imaging tools have become alternative noninvasive detection tools that can be routinely employed in clinical practice. The NAFLD activity score is important as part of the diagnosis procedure. But the fibrosis score is just as important. **Table 2** shows the fibrosis score currently used to stage the degree of fibrosis in the liver. There are a few noninvasive fibrosis imaging tests on the market such as Fibroscan that offers a liver stiffness measurement (LSM) using pulsed-echo ultrasound as a surrogate marker of fibrosis [70] and acoustic radiation force impulse (ARFI), which uses conventional B-mode ultrasonography to produce an ultrasonic pulse and measure the response of the liver tissue as shear wave velocity [71]. The Centers for Disease Control (CDC) and Prevention projects that diabetes mellitus is likely to impact the fibrosis progression rates, given the close link between diabetes and fibrosis in those with NAFLD [72, 73].

Some commercial biomarker tests include enhanced liver fibrosis (ELF), a panel of markers of matrix turnover as tissue inhibitor of matrix metalloproteinase 1 (TIMP1), hyaluronic acid and PIIINP [74] and FibroTest (FT), a panel of markers of fibrosis widely used in France.

Grade	Steatosis (%)	S score	Lobular (L) inflammation	L score	Hepatocyte ballooning (B)	B score
0	<5	0	No foci	0	None	0
1	5–33	1	<2 foci per 200 × field	1	Few cells	1
2	34–66	2	2–4 foci per 200 × filed	2	Many cells	2
3	>66	3	>4 foci per 200 × filed	3	N/A	N/A

NASH activity grade = total score: S + L + B range (0–8). Score of ≥5 is equivalent to NASH; score of 3 or 4 is borderline NASH; score of ≤2 denotes non-NASH NAFLD. The NAFLD activity score is based on three pathologic features: Steatosis, hepatocyte ballooning degeneration, and lobular inflammation. Higher scoring denotes severity of NASH: >5 = NASH; <5 = No NASH; 3–4 = borderline; none (0); few (1); many (2).

Table 1.
NAFLD activity score (NAS).

Liver injury	Fibrosis score (0–4)*	Fibrosis stage
None	0	0
Mild (delicate fibrosis)/zone 3 presinusoidal fibrosis	<5% (0), 5–33% = (1)	1a
Moderate (dense fibrosis)/zone 3 presinusoidal fibrosis	>33–66% (2), >66% = (3)	1b
Periportal/portal fibrosis	0 (0), <2 (1), 2–4 (2), > (3)	1c
Portal and periportal fibrosis/presinusoidal fibrosis	None (0)	2
Bridging fibrosis	Few (1)	3
Cirrhosis	Many (2)	4

**Fibrosis score of F1-F4 is generally considered NASH [4].*

Table 2.
NAFLD fibrosis score (NFS) and stage.

1.4 The metabolic syndrome (MetS)

Recognizing patients with the metabolic syndrome (MetS) is key to identifying patients at risk of NAFLD. MetS is a group of risk factors that raises risk of heart disease, diabetes, stroke, etc. [75] and is diagnosed when any three of the following five clinical risk factors are present [76]: impaired fasting serum glucose, low levels of serum HDL cholesterol, elevated serum triglycerides (i.e., hypertriglyceridemia), central obesity or larger than cut-off waist circumference (varies according to gender and ethnicity), and high blood pressure (HTN) (see **Table 3**).

Insulin resistance is also a major risk factor for the development of steatosis. Once considered benign, NAFL (or simple steatosis), which is defined as the presence of hepatic steatosis with no evidence of hepatocellular injury in the form of ballooning of the hepatocytes, is now believed to be a serious risk factor for progression to liver disease, cardiovascular disease, and mortality [37, 77]. This is because an excess of abdominal fat is most tightly associated with the metabolic risk factors [78, 79]. The duration of obesity and the presence of MetS in an individual patient are closely tied to the risk of developing NASH-related cirrhosis and HCC [80]. Some of the characteristics of MetS are present in most NAFLD individuals, with 65–71% being obese, 57–68% having deranged lipid profiles, 36–70% suffering from HTN, and 12–37% having impaired fasting glucose tolerance [81]. Approximately a third of patients with NAFLD have the full metabolic syndrome and >90% have at least one feature [47]. There is a consensus that considers NAFLD as a hepatic manifestation of the MetS [82, 83]. On the other hand, clinical signs of the disease are manifested in 70–75% of T2DM patients and up to 95% of obese patients [84]. Thus, the development of the MetS, which is an important

Features	Terms of condition
Blood glucose (sugar)	Fasting, ≥100 mg/dL
Blood HDL ("good") cholesterol	♂ < 40 mg/dL; ♀ < 50 mg/dL
Blood triglycerides (TGs)	Fasting, ≥150 mg/dL
Waist circumference	♂ > 40″; ♀ > 35″
Blood pressure (HTN)	≥130/85 mm Hg

**The MetS is present with any three of the features shown in the table.*
♂ = male; ♀ = female; HDL = high-density lipoprotein; ″ = inches.

Table 3.
*Features of the metabolic syndrome.**

predictor of NASH in NAFLD patients, poses a sweeping and unfavorable prognosis [85]. IR is a key mediator that links NAFLD and MetS, which is a constellation of anthropometric and metabolic abnormalities (see **Table 3** above).

According to the latest data from NHANES (National Health and Nutrition Examination Survey) study conducted between 2011 and 2012, the prevalence of MetS has increased to 35% in American adults [86]. MetS is a risk factor for diabetes and cardiovascular diseases. It induces an abnormal production of hormones such as leptin, adiponectin, and cytokines such as TNF (tumor necrosis factor)-alpha that regulate inflammatory responses and cause disequilibrium between the pro-inflammatory and anti-inflammatory state of the organ [86]. These are mutually antagonistic: the pro-inflammatory factors such as TNF-alpha promote pro-apoptotic processes, recruit white blood cells, and promote insulin resistance. On the other hand, adiponectin acting as an anti-inflammatory factor inhibits fatty acid uptake, stimulates fatty acid oxidation and lipid export, and enhances insulin sensitivity. Both an increase in pro-inflammatory factors and a decrease in anti-inflammatory factors cause a cytokine imbalance that would lead to steatosis (NAFL) followed by necroinflammation (NASH) and IR. There is a supporting evidence that a high TNF to adiponectin ratio promotes fatty liver and steatohepatitis in animal [87] and human [88] studies. The importance of MetS including IR is that it predicts the occurrence of diabetes and cardiovascular diseases, which can further promote the development and progression of arteriosclerosis and HTN leading to significant morbidity and mortality [89]. Also, NAFLD and obesity are risk factors for the progression to fibrosis among HCV-infected patients [90–93]. Furthermore, elevated levels of ferritin are common in NAFLD patients and typically reflect active IR or underlying inflammatory activity [68, 81, 94]. Therefore, because of many different correlates and etiological factors and an assortment of assessment tools associated with MetS, there are some unresolved uncertainties in the current estimates of the global and the United States prevalence of NAFLD.

1.5 The genetics of NAFLD

Genetic disorders of lipid metabolism can cause hepatic fat deposition. However, they are far less common than excess body weight and features of MetS as risk factors for NAFLD and NASH. Several genes have been associated with NAFLD. These include *NCAN*, which may have a protective effect for Hispanics but increases risk of steatosis for non-Hispanic blacks; *LYPLAL1*, *GCKR*, as well as *PPP1R3B*, which may confer increased risk for hepatic steatosis but the data of distinctive serum lipid profiles in all these genes are sparse [61, 95–97]. *GCKR* is reported to be closely associated with NAFLD in Chinese [98]. Another gene, Patatin-like phospholipase domain-containing 3 (*PNPLA3* or adiponutrin), has emerged as the genetic factor predisposing Hispanics more at risk for fatty liver disease [99]. This adiponutrin gene is a single variant considered responsible for increased hepatic TG levels, fibrosis, and inflammation, observed among ethnic groups [100, 101]. Homozygote patients have a twofold rise in hepatic fat content than heterozygotes, and Hispanic populations exhibit the highest frequency of this polymorphism (49%) compared to 23% in European-Americans (EAs) and 17% in African-Americans (AAs) [101]. It also shows more allelic frequency with Hispanics than other ethnic groups. Romeo and colleagues [102, 103] along with Singal and colleagues published papers in 2008 in which they reported that *PNPLA3* is strongly associated with hepatic steatosis and elevated ALT and also recently showed that *PNPLA3* is associated with NASH, fibrosis progression, and hepatocellular cancer as well [102].

A genetic marker, *TM6SF2*, discovered in an exome-wide association study of liver fat content, has also shed some light on its association with hepatic steatosis. It is involved in the loss of function mutation in very low-density lipoprotein (VLDL) secretion, and its association with NASH and advanced fibrosis has been recently validated even though its precise function has not been delineated [102]. However, its mutation is associated with elevated ALT, hepatic steatosis, and lower level of alkaline phosphatase, LDL, and TGs. This gene is most prevalent in European ancestry and less in Hispanics and AAs [104].

There is a reported 52% heritability rate of NAFLD, but evidence pertaining to specific genetic mutations is scant according to multivariable models used after adjusting for sex, age, and ethnicity [13]. Although the mechanism is not well understood, genetic mutations in hemochromatosis (HFE) gene, which is responsible for iron uptake and transferrin plasma concentration, may also be associated with NAFLD development [105, 106]. Several other factors have been indicated in the development and outcomes of NAFLD including epigenetic alterations [107, 108], maternal perinatal nutrition [109–111], and gut microbiota [107, 112–114]. A recent study also reports a novel pathway in which hepatic vitamin D receptor (VDR) expression is increased in patients with simple steatosis (nonalcoholic fatty liver without inflammation), and the activated VDR upregulates angiopoietin-like protein 8 (ANGPTL8) expression, thus contributing to triglyceride accumulation in human hepatocytes [115]. At any rate, studies have reported that fibrosis-initiated fatty liver disease progresses over many years, thus providing a potential window for intervention by examining disease-progression/modifying factors in NAFLD [116–118]. It is important to note that increased BMI and insulin resistance have been associated with a more rapid progression to fibrosis [35, 119].

1.6 The epidemiology and prevalence of NAFLD

In most epidemiological studies, the prevalence of NAFLD in the general population is determined by imaging or other indirect methods. Accordingly, the epidemiology and demographic characteristics of NAFLD vary worldwide [12, 16]. In epidemiological studies, the pathophysiological aspects, the natural history, and the determinants of NAFLD are important parameters for the diagnosis and evaluation of therapeutic interventions. This section will provide global perspectives on the prevalence of NAFLD (and later HCC) with emphasis on the United States and the possible reasons for the rapid rise.

There are wide-ranging estimates of NAFLD prevalence in the general population of the United States. An estimated 17–51% of adults have NAFLD [23, 120, 121]. Analysis of liver ultrasound data collected between 1988 and 1994 from the NHANES III reported that 19% of adults have NAFLD [122], whereas a meta-analysis of studies from 2006 to 2014 estimated a NAFLD prevalence of 24% (20–29%) in the general population [65]. The prevalence of NASH is difficult to estimate as biopsy is the necessary tool for screening, but it is cost-prohibitive and impractical for a population study.

Globally, NAFLD is a growing cause of chronic liver disease and NASH is replacing HCV infection as the primary reason for LT [13, 123, 124]. The broad category of NAFLD can manifest as NAFL or NASH. Fibrosis precedes cirrhosis and is therefore used as a prognosticator of the clinical risk of progression to cirrhosis and long-term liver-related adverse outcomes and mortality [34]. Recent evidence has shown that NAFLD and NASH can progress to HCC even in the absence of cirrhosis [125–127]. In most epidemiological studies including the NHANES data set, the assumptions about NASH in the NAFLD population are based on a post-hoc application of liver enzymes (i.e., AST and ALT) and clinical measurements. In the same vein, the fibrosis stages in population-based studies reflect best estimates derived from clinical aids (e.g., fibrosis-4, ALT to platelet ratio index, and NAFLD fibrosis scores) [128, 129]. The current prevalence rates for NAFLD, NASH, and HCC based on definitive clinical manifestations are shown in **Table 4**.

Certain risk factors such as advanced age, obesity, ethnicity, and T2DM increase the incidence and prevalence of NAFLD and NASH and have been consistently identified as salient risk factors for fibrotic progression to cirrhosis [130] (see **Table 5**).

The current global estimate is that 24–30% of the world's population is affected by NAFLD [65] and that includes between 80 and 100 million Americans (http://www.mayoclinic.com), making it the primary etiology for liver disease in the United States; see **Figure 2**.

The increasing incidence of obesity, diabetes, and metabolic syndrome in the United States and Europe may soon catapult NAFLD/NASH to become the most common cause of HCC in developed countries. In the United States, among the more than 26 million people with diabetes, the prevalence of biopsy-proven NAFLD and NASH is as high as 74 and 11%, respectively [138, 139].

1.7 The rise in burden of NAFLD/NASH

The global rise of NAFLD has exasperated the looming healthcare burden of disease. It may be difficult to accurately forecast the current and future burden of a disease that is rapidly progressing. However, there are modeling techniques and approaches that incorporate real-world surveillance data for NAFLD and NASH incidences, which are growing causes of cirrhosis and HCC. As with many models, the utility of the model is linked to the validity of the inputs into the model. One of these modeling approaches is based on the premise that public awareness and

Status	Definition	Prevalence	Prognosis
NAFLD	Spectrum of fatty liver disease with <140 g for men and < 70 g for women per week of alcohol consumption	Estimated at 24–30% of global population [13, 14, 16] and at least 31% of US population (7)	—
NAFL	>5% simple hepatic steatosis by weight of liver without evidence of hepatocellular injury (i.e., hepatocyte ballooning)	>80% of NAFLD patients	Low probability of progression to cirrhosis
NASH	>5% hepatic steatosis by weight of liver with inflammation and hepatocellular injury with or without fibrosis Confirmed histologically	Estimated at up to 21–59% of patients with NAFLD Estimated at 1.5–6.45% of US general US population [40, 96, 122]	11% progress to cirrhosis over 15 years
NASH cirrhosis	Presence of cirrhosis with current or past histologic evidence of steatosis	10–30% of patients with NASH	About 31% have liver decompensation over 8 years; about 7% develop HCC over 6.5 years
NASH HCC	Hepatocellular carcinoma induced by NASH	Estimated at annual rate of 2.6–12.8%*	Progresses to end-stage liver disease

**The prevalence of NASH-HCC is not firmly established. Data in the table are the annual incidence rate of developing HCC in patients with NASH-related cirrhosis.*

Table 4.
Prevalence of NAFLD and its more progressive forms, NASH and HCC.

Risk factor	Description	References
Age	Risk increases with age	[4, 40]
Gender	More common in men Higher risk of advanced fibrosis in women	[4, 96, 131, 132]
Genetics	Patatin-like phospholipase domain-containing 3 gene	[133]
MetS**	70–90% of patients have NAFLD MetS is an independent predictor of fibrosis	[85, 95]
Ethnicity	Elevated risk in Hispanics Lower risk in blacks	[61]
Diet	Elevated levels of cholesterol and saturated fats High fructose intake, low carbohydrates	[89, 134–136]
OSA***	Increased risk of hepatic fibrosis	[137]

**NAFLD/NASH = nonalcoholic fatty liver disease/nonalcoholic steatohepatitis.*
***MetS = metabolic syndrome.*
****OSA = obstructive sleep apnea.*

Table 5.
NAFLD/NASH risk factors.*

government health policies will be able to eventually level off national obesity incidences and prevalence, which in return will level off NAFLD [4]. The interpretation of the output of this and other models attempting to analyze the burden of NAFLD is constrained by the lack of accurate diagnosis of steatohepatitis with simple epidemiologic tools. Nevertheless, the proportion of individuals with NASH in the NAFLD population will probably continue to rise through the next 15 years based on the rising prevalence of diabetes mellitus [4].

Analyzing the cost and burden of disease with respect to NASH has several potential implications. First, it helps introduce strategies and treatment regimen that will stem its exponential rise in incidence and mortality rates; it will reduce the growing contribution of NASH to LT, which is expensive; and due to an oversupply of decompensated cirrhosis, matching organ availability is rare, and insurance companies have exclusive policy of qualifying subjects with NASH-induced cirrhosis based on whether they have associated co-morbidities.

The epidemiology and demographic characteristics of NAFLD vary worldwide. The rise in NAFLD and NASH will balloon the number of patients with decompensated cirrhosis and pose a major emotional and financial burden on subjects and

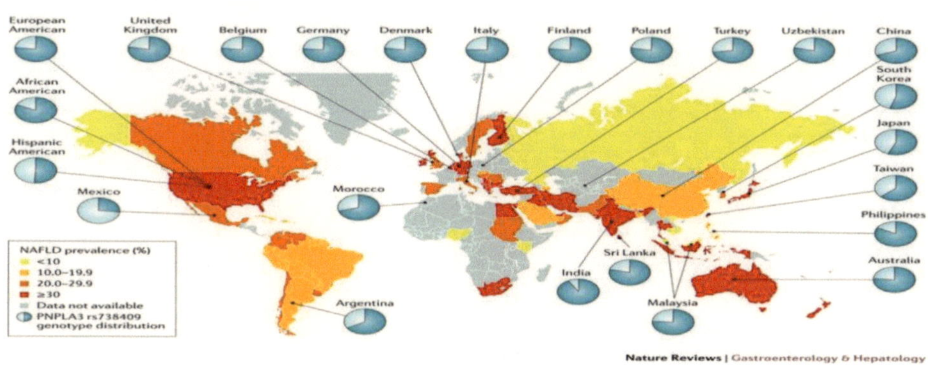

Figure 2.
Global picture of estimated prevalence of NAFLD and distribution of PNPLA3 genotypes adopted from Zobair Younossi [16]. PNPLA3 is presented as minor allele frequency in some areas (light blue section of the pie chart).

their caregivers, thus adding to the overall cost of health care. Furthermore, the main etiologic factor adding to the burden of HCC is NAFLD [4]. In select NASH-related HCC patients, liver resection and transplantation provide potentially curative therapeutic options; however, these procedures place a significant burden to health-care resources and utilization [140]. Currently, NASH-related HCC has replaced HCV-related HCC as the fastest growing indication for LT in HCC candidates.

2. Hepatocellular carcinoma (HCC)

Liver cancer, which has limited therapeutic choices, has the second highest mortality rate in the world [141]. HCC, which can lead to complications such as portal vein thrombosis (PVT), accounts for the majority of primary liver malignancies and is one of the leading causes of death in patients with advanced fibrosis or cirrhosis [141–144]. HCC can be caused by chronic infection with hepatitis B virus (HBV) or hepatitis C virus (HCV), alcohol abuse, as well as obesity and diabetes-induced MetS. NAFLD often occurs in the setting of metabolic disorders such as obesity and T2DM. These same metabolic conditions are also risk factors for NAFLD-associated HCC, which can materialize in individuals even in the absence of advanced fibrosis or cirrhosis. NASH-HCC appears to be phenotypically different from HCC arising from other chronic liver diseases (**Table 6**). By all accounts, the formation and progression of HCC are multistep processes. Therefore, the specific and detailed molecular events that underlie HCC development remain only partially understood [143].

2.1 The epidemiology and prevalence of HCC

Primary liver cancer in 2012 was identified as the second most common cause of cancer-related death in the world. In the United States, HCC is the most common histological subtype of liver cancer that accounts for 70–85% of primary liver malignancies [145, 146]. It is also the most rapidly rising cause of cancer and

Hepatitis B infection (HBV)
Hepatitis C infection (HCV)
Hepatitis D infection (HDV)
Alcohol (ethanol)
Nonalcoholic fatty liver disease (NAFLD)/nonalcoholic steatohepatitis (NASH)
Obesity/diabetes
Hereditary hemochromatosis
Aflatoxin B
Tyrosinemia
Glycogen storage disease type 1a
Oral contraceptives
Smoking
Cirrhosis*

**Diagnosis of cirrhosis is based on the presence of the ICD-9 codes for cirrhosis or complications of cirrhosis (gastroesophageal varices, encephalopathy, and nonmalignant ascites) recorded at least twice in any inpatient or outpatient encounter.*

Table 6.
Common risk factors for hepatocellular carcinoma.

cancer-related deaths with an incidence that has more than tripled over the last two decades. This high mortality reflects a poor prognosis and a poorer therapeutic intervention [147]. Compared to HCC caused by alcoholic liver disease and viral hepatitis, there is a lack of strong epidemiological data associated with the incidence and prevalence of HCC precipitating from NAFLD [140, 148]. While the prevalence of NAFLD is thought to be highest among Hispanics and Caucasians, the ethnic distribution among NAFLD-/NASH-related HCC patients has yet to be defined. Male patients are overrepresented in NASH-related HCC; however, gender has not been proven to be a statistical risk factor in NASH progression to HCC [7]. The rising incidence of NAFLD/NASH in the setting of obesity has led to a drastic growth in NASH-related HCC incidence [149]. Although NAFLD can present with HCC in the absence of NASH or cirrhosis, the cumulative annual incidence rate for developing HCC in patients with NASH-related cirrhosis is approximately 2.4–12.8% [125]. This suggests or utmost underlies that cirrhosis may be the main cause of HCC despite new emerging data suggesting that NAFLD may be an independent risk factor for HCC, even in the absence of cirrhosis [126, 150, 151].

There was also a twofold increase in the incidence of HCC in the United States over the past two decades, and it is projected to double over the next two decades. Compared to HCC in alcoholic liver disease and viral hepatitis, there is a lack of strong epidemiological data regarding the incidence and prevalence of HCC in NAFLD [148]. It is projected that in just 12 more years, HCC at its current pace of growth in the United States will outstrip breast and colorectal cancers as the third leading cause of cancer-related death. This is because the prevalence of HCC is expected to increase by 149% from 10,000 to 24,900 during 2015–2030, while the incidence of HCC cases is expected to increase from 5160 to 12,240 in 2030, an increase of 137% [4]. This alarming incidence is attributed to several different genetic and epigenetic alterations that are under investigation [4].

Modeling the epidemic of HCC suggests that in 2015, 3280 incident HCC cases were estimated to have progressed from compensated cirrhosis (64% of total), with the remaining 1880 incident cases occurring among ≤F3 (fibrosis score-3) cases [4]. By 2030, 8790 incident HCC cases are predicted to occur among compensated cirrhotic cases or 72% of the annual incidence, reflecting aging and disease progression [4].

The true prevalence of NASH and NASH-related HCC is probably underestimated. This is because in 6.9–29% of HCC cases, the underlying etiology is unknown, further questioning the designation that the liver disease is secondary to cryptogenic cirrhosis [148]. Traits of NASH are more frequently observed in HCC patients with cryptogenic cirrhosis than in age- and sex-matched HCC patients of well-defined viral or alcoholic etiology [152]. In the past several years, myriad studies have tried to determine the variability of relationships between NAFLD/NASH, cryptogenic cirrhosis, and HCC. In a recent meta-analysis, White et al. [125] estimated that 60% of HCC cases ascribed to NAFLD/NASH had cirrhosis either prior to diagnosis or at the time of diagnosis. This same analysis showed that NASH-associated cirrhosis consistently manifested an increased HCC risk. Furthermore, the study also revealed that when compared to those with chronic HCV, the risk of developing HCC is lower in patients with cirrhosis due to NAFLD/NASH (HCV, 19.7% vs. NAFLD/NASH, 26.9%) [125]. Although the prevalence of NAFLD-/NASH-related HCC is not well delineated, the growing incidence of obesity and diabetes suggests the impact of NAFLD-/NASH-related HCC will continue to grow.

2.2 The genetics of HCC

Genomic analyses promise to improve tumor characterization for the optimization of precision or personalized medicine for patients with HCC. Recent developments and molecular techniques have significantly improved our understanding of the pathogenesis of HCC and its complex genetic landscape [153–156]. The integration of several profiling data from various sources may provide additional insight into the molecular mechanisms of HCC [153]. The first large-scale multiplatform analysis of HCC conducted as part of The Cancer Genome Atlas (TCGA) network included valuation of somatic mutations by whole exome sequencing and DNA copy number analyses in 363 patients whose tissue and tumor specimens were obtained [157]. This high-throughput analysis also included further investigation of DNA methylation, mRNA expression, microRNA (miRNA) expression, and proteomic expression in 196 patients. To decipher the molecular landscape of HCC and extract biological insights for therapeutic targets and prognostic implications, analyses were made by integrating multiple data platforms with the available clinical data for HCC [157]. Mutational and DNA sequencing analyses identified an array of genes altered either by downregulation or by mutation. Among the significantly mutated genes were EEF1A1, SMARCA4, LZTR1, and SF3B1 [157]. Those genes downregulated by hypermethylation including ALB, APOB, and CPS1 may cause metabolic reprogramming in HCC. The analysis of integrated molecular platform also yielded the identification of a subtype linked to poorer prognosis in three HCC cohorts. This large-scale multiplatform, high-throughput analysis enabled the design of a p53 target gene expression signature correlating with poor survival. This TCGA network analysis produced potential therapeutic targets including WNT signaling, IDH1, MET, VEGFA, MCL1, MDM4, TERT, and immune checkpoint proteins PD-1, PD-L1, and CTLA-4 [157]. This is significant because effective inhibitors already exit for these targets, which alter hepatocyte energy balance [157].

In exome sequencing analysis of over 200 liver tumors, investigators identified mutational signatures that are associated with specific risk factors such as alcohol and tobacco consumption and exposure to aflatoxin B_1 [158]. As a result, they found that 161 putative driver genes were associated with 11 recurrently altered pathways involving *CTNNB1* (alcohol), *TP53* (hepatitis B virus, HBV), and *AXIN1* [158]. Further analysis of tumor stage progression identified *TERT* as an early event, whereas *FGF3*, *FGF4*, *FGF19*, or *CCND1* amplification and *TP53* and *CDKN2A* alterations were prominent in aggressive tumors. The involvement of these many altered genes and pathways in the development and/or progression of HCC leads to the extensive landscape and multifaceted nature of this lethal cancer. **Figure 3** shows the salient signaling pathways associated with HCC.

In another recent study, gene expression and DNA methylation profiles were screened to identify potential genetic biomarkers of HCC. The findings from this study suggest potential HCC biomarker roles for certain genes such as *DTL, DUSP1, NFKBIA*, and *SOCS2* [160]. Similar to TCGA Research Network analyses mentioned above [157], these investigators also suggest that the tumor protein 'p53 signaling' and 'metabolic' pathways may serve important roles in the pathogenesis of HCC [160]. Other polymorphic variants serving as potential risk factors for HCC in high-risk patients infected with HBV/HCV have also been reported [161]. As for prognostic biomarkers, recent RNA sequencing data from the Cancer Genome Atlas (TCGA) reveal that among the 12 tissue types studied, the liver had the largest number of tissue-enriched genes, which are associated with the prognosis of patients with HCC and represent distinct physiological patterns [162]. A further study of the characteristics of liver-enriched genes showed that hypermethylation might be partially responsible for the downregulation of these genes, most of which were metabolism-related genes associated with pathological stage and dedifferentiation in patients with HCC. The authors suggest that hypermethylation might be a mechanism

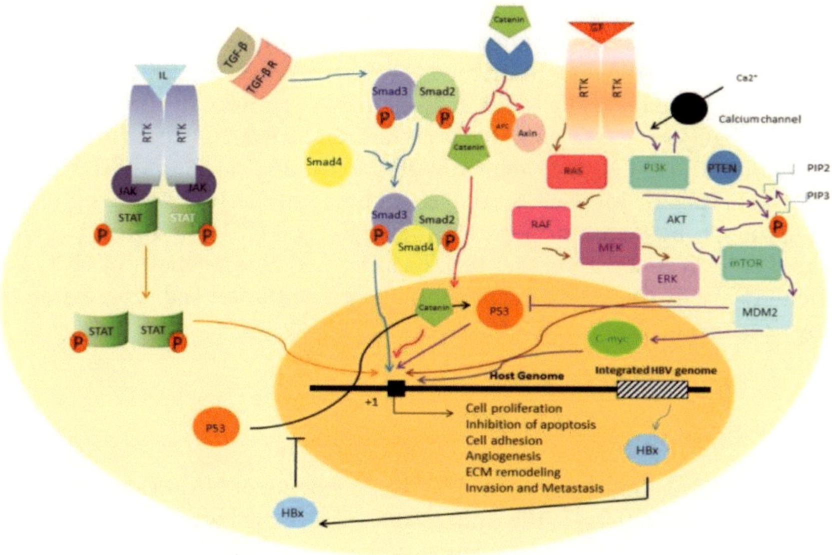

Figure 3.
The most reported signaling pathways in HCC. Adapted from Birgani et al. [159].

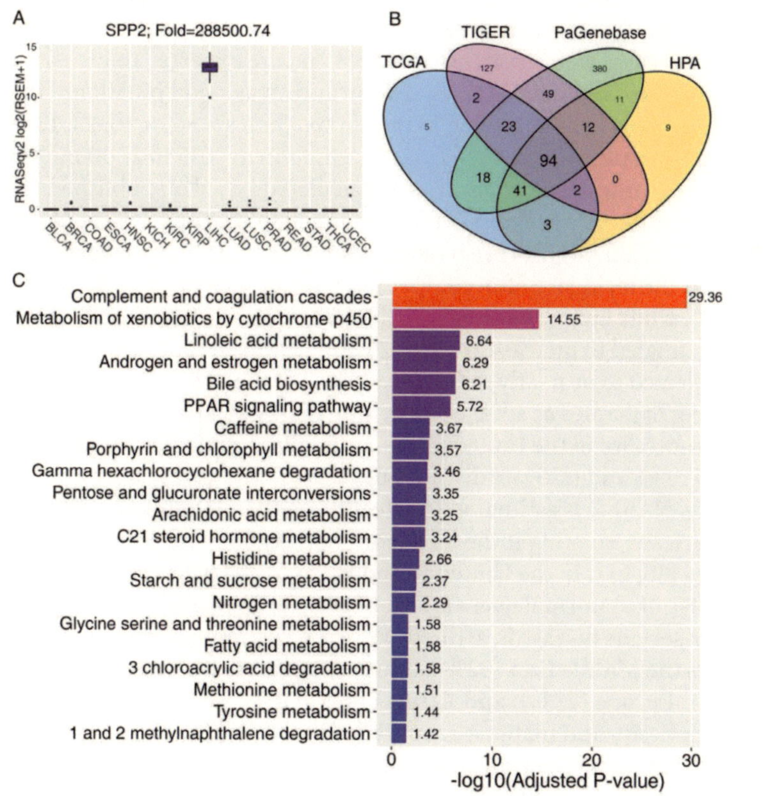

Figure 4.
Validation of liver-enriched genes and KEGG analysis. (A) an example of liver-enriched genes. SPP2 was exclusively expressed in the corresponding nontumor tissues of HCC. (B) Four-set Venn diagram showing the overlap of the liver-enriched genes derived from the TCGA and three other databases, including HPA, PaGenBase, and TiGER. (C) Significantly enriched KEGG pathways of 188 liver-enriched genes. −log10 (adjusted p-value) was annotated on each bar of the KEGG pathway. Adapted from Binghua et al. [162].

underlying the downregulation of these liver-enriched genes. When they overlapped the tissue-enriched and prognostic genes across cancer types, they found that, in HCC, 55% (84/188) of the liver-enriched genes were prognostic (see **Figure 4**).

Circulating regulatory nucleic acids like miRNA profiles can also reflect the pathogenic changes occurring in organs including the liver. Changes in miR-21, miR-122, and miR-223 were correlated with the histological status of the human liver and were specific for liver injury [163]. These miRNA levels were significantly higher in the serum of chronic hepatitis (i.e., HBV and HCV) and HCC patients compared to healthy controls [44]. Yet, the biological heterogeneity of HCC makes it difficult to clarify the key mechanisms of cancer initiation and progression, and thereby develop and implement effective therapies [164].

3. The projection of NAFLD and HCC

A recent Markov model was used to predict incidence of NAFLD and to forecast NAFLD disease progression in the United States. The model was based on historical and projected changes in adult prevalence of obesity and T2DM as well as national surveillance data for incidence of NAFLD-related HCC [4]. The report forecasts that prevalent NAFLD cases will increase to 21% (100.9 million) by 2030, while prevalent NASH cases will increase 63% from 16.5 million to 27.00 million cases [4]. Overall NAFLD prevalence among the adult population (aged ≥15 years) is projected at 33.5% in 2030, and the median age of the NAFLD population will increase from 50 (estimated at 2015 level) to 55 years between 2015 and 2030 [4]. In 2015, approximately 20% of NAFLD cases were classified as NASH and are expected to increase to 27% by 2030, a reflection of both disease progression and an aging population. The estimated prevalence of NASH in adults living in the United States is 3–5% [6, 23, 121, 165] and is projected to increase by 63% from 16.5 million in 2015 to 27.00 million cases in 2030 [4]. This prevalence of NASH was calculated based on published estimates and modeling of fibrosis progression. It was assumed that up to 5% of NAFLD cases without NASH could be NASH regressors, with most NASH regressors still in F0 stage [4]. Similarly, the incidence of decompensated cirrhosis will surge by 168% to 105,430 cases in 2030, while incidence of HCC will increase by 137% to 12,240 cases. Liver deaths are estimated to increase 178% to 78,300 deaths in 2030. During 2015–2030, there are projected to be nearly 800,000 excess liver deaths. The aging population, the continuing high rates of adult obesity, and T2DM will propel NAFLD-related liver disease and mortality in the United States. Immediate strategies are required to curtail new NAFLD cases and mitigate disease burden.

Currently, NAFLD is estimated to affect more than 80 million and up to 90 million Americans, making it the most common etiology for liver disease in the United States [16, 65]. In the United Kingdom, NAFLD has now become the most common cause of abnormal liver function tests (LFTs) [166]. Although NAFLD has emerged as a serious disease in affluent Western economies, its global prevalence encompasses the Middle East (32%), South America (31%), Asia (27%), the United States (24%), Europe (23%), and Africa (14%) [167]. Because of the increasing incidence of obesity and diabetes around the world, NAFLD has become a global public health concern. The prevalence of NAFLD varies according to age, sex, and the methodology used to measure the condition in each geographical location [61]. Currently, NAFLD is the most prevalent liver disease observed in patients with obesity, diabetes, and metabolic syndrome (MetS), all of which can confer insulin resistance (IR) and are known risk factors for the development of HCC, a growing indicator of LT [45, 69]. While HCV infection has been the most common indication for liver transplants to date, NASH is surpassing it as obesity reaches historic

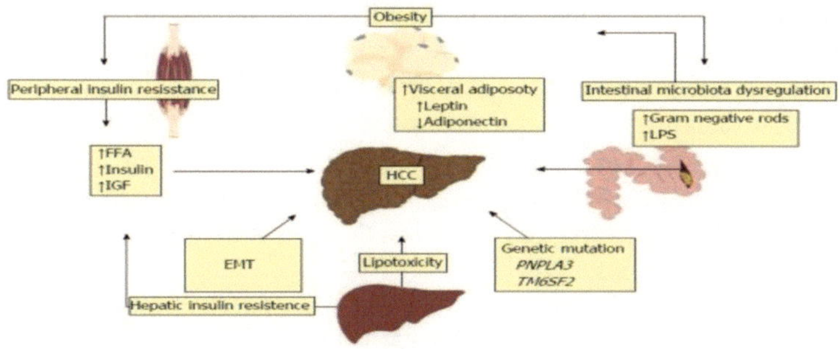

Figure 5.
Risk factors and proposed mechanisms for NAFLD- and NASH-related HCC, which is multifactorial. Proposed pathogenic mechanisms include obesity, peripheral and hepatic IR from T2DM, increased hepatic lipid storage and lipotoxicity, genetic mutations, and intestinal microbiota dysregulation. HCC, hepatocellular carcinoma; EMT, epithelial to mesenchymal transition; NAFLD, nonalcoholic fatty liver disease; NASH, nonalcoholic steatohepatitis; FFA, free fatty acid; IGF, insulin-like growth factor; LPS, lipopolysaccharide; PNPLA3, *patatin-like phospholipase domain-containing 3; TM6SF2, transmembrane 6 superfamily member 2. Adapted from Cholankeril [140].*

highs and new direct-acting antiviral (DAA) drugs are essentially curing hepatitis C [168]. Furthermore, with the continued decline in the prevalence of HCV infection, the proportion of NASH-HCC is anticipated to increase exponentially due to the growing epidemic of obesity and diabetes [140]. Currently, NASH-related HCC is the fastest growing indication for LT in HCC candidates [140]. NAFLD and NASH are a growing cause of cirrhosis and HCC.

Globally, Asia is leading the rise in NAFLD followed by the United States. Although our understanding of NAFLD is steadily evolving, it is not an isolated disease. It is commonly associated with the leading metabolic comorbidities such as obesity, MetS, T2DM, and dyslipidemia. The potential progression of NAFLD subtypes is from fibrosis to advanced fibrosis, ESLD, and HCC (**Figure 1**). As the incidence of obesity and concurrently diabetes and MetS continues to surge in Europe and the United States, NAFLD/NASH may become the most common cause of HCC in developed countries in the foreseeable future [169–171].

A 2002–2012 retrospective cohort study among adult patients revealed a fourfold increase in patients undergoing LT for NASH-related HCC in contrast to only twofold increase in number of patients undergoing transplantation for HCV-related HCC. In the United States, about 6000–7000 liver transplants are performed annually, and the rapid increase in the percentage (44.9%) of obese individuals during a 14-year period (2000–2014) is expected to escalate to 55% the number of NASH patients awaiting LT by 2030 [172]. The increased morbidity and mortality, healthcare costs, and declining health-related quality of life associated with NAFLD require more in-depth analysis. **Figure 5** depicts the proposed mechanisms that ties NAFLD/NASH and HCC.

4. Ethnic and gender differences in NAFLD and HCC

Although still not fully resolved, the prevalence of NAFLD in the United States can vary by ethnicity. Even in this context, there are several factors that could explain the reported ethnic disparities. These include access to health care, genetic factors, environmental factors, affliction with chronic diseases, and the presence of chronic diseases such as the MetS [61, 65, 173]. In this context, the prevalence of NAFLD is reported to be highest in Hispanic-Americans, followed by Americans of European descent and then African-Americans [40, 61, 65, 122, 173]. Several studies have shown a relative sparsity of NAFLD cases among individuals of African descent living in or coming from Africa or the Caribbean region. Although the prevalence of metabolic disease and obesity is high in Afro-Caribbean ethnic groups compared to Caucasian and Hispanic groups, the frequency of NAFLD/NASH is reported to be low [61, 174]. This discrepancy might be due to an actual low number rate or biases that include low-recognition and low-referral rates in these ethnic minorities [175], as Afro-Caribbean patients are categorically less likely to be referred to other tertiary hospitals [176].

There are also ethnic differences in the incidence of HCC in the United States (see Sherif et al. for a comprehensive review) [61]. Compared to European-Americans (EAs), the incidence of HCC is higher in African-Americans (AAs) and is associated with more advanced tumor stage at diagnosis and lower survival rates overall. Assessment of changes in the levels of metabolites of samples stratified by race was made using gas chromatography-mass spectrometry in selected ion monitoring mode to identify ethnically diverse biomarkers in HCC between EA and AAs [177]. Race-specific metabolites including alpha tocopherol for AA and EA combined, glycine for EA, and valine for AA exhibited better sensitivity and specificity than the standard serological marker for HCC, alpha-fetoprotein (AFP) that is widely used for the diagnosis of HCC [177–180]. It is hypothesized that there is a variation in HCC-associated epigenetic modifications between AAs and EAs. Thus, the identification of aberrant DNA methylation and differentially modulated miRNAs can be used to better understand the mechanisms of disparities in HCC between races. Also, identifying epigenetic markers for HCC in a specific population will enhance personalized medicine that targets specific therapeutic approaches [181, 182]. This also demands the gathering together of a highly interdisciplinary team of experts to investigate changes in both DNA methylation and miRNA expression patterns between tumor, cirrhotic, and normal liver tissues from AA and EA participants. Identifying molecular cancer gene drivers and mutations may 1 day become critical for precision oncology.

Most epidemiological studies document prevalence of individual diseases in selected tertiary hospital populations [183]. This widespread practice, particularly when imaging and liver enzyme tests are involved and when the patients may be asymptomatic in the early stage of diagnosis, leads to underestimation and underdiagnosis of NAFLD. This is especially true for minority populations in whom the natural development and progression of NAFLD and NASH are understudied and underreported as reflected by the paucity of data in the literature. Furthermore, the predictive value of the MetS may not reflect the true state of NAFLD in AAs since the criteria for the syndrome were developed for non-Hispanic whites [184] thereby influencing underdiagnosis or misdiagnosis of NAFLD and NASH in Hispanics and non-Hispanic blacks (NHB). There is also a strong relationship between insulin resistance and hypertriglyceridemia, one of the crucial components of MetS. However, NHB often have normal triglycerides (TG) level [185], which is used as a diagnostic criterion of the MetS leading to underdiagnosis of the MetS in NHB [186]. This suggests that lowering the threshold for TG level in AAs will lead to grasping the true cases of NAFLD. Moreover, the racial differences in NAFLD and NASH may be a function of the differences in TGs or the differences in the distribution of adiposity (e.g., subcutaneous vs. visceral) since AAs have relatively less VAT and lower TGs than Hispanics [119, 173, 175]. In addition, AAs may be more resistant to both the accretion of TG in the abdominal visceral compartment (adipose tissue and liver) and hypertriglyceridemia associated with IR [119].

Epidemiologic studies establish the foundational framework for the control and prevention of diseases. In the case of NAFLD and NASH, it should be done by first tracking the prevalence of the disease, characterizing its natural history, and identifying both its social and health determinants along ethnic lines. This type of study is critical for the proper diagnosis and early intervention of NAFLD especially in minority populations [61].

Genome-wide association studies have revealed several genetic variants that are associated with NAFLD and NASH. Yet, these variants either represent only a limited amount of variation in hepatic steatosis among ethnic groups or may just be markers representing a larger body of genetic variations.

There is an urgent need to gain a better understanding of the underlying biological mechanisms responsible for why some people with NAFLD are more prone to developing HCC, and the causes for disparities in NAFLD-related HCC. There is also an urgent need for a less invasive method than biopsy and for a more sensitive biomarker than ALT for large-scale NAFLD screening. The lack of high-throughput studies employing proteomics or metabolomics for the discovery of novel and reliable diagnostic biomarkers for NAFLD also hampers our understanding of the pathophysiology of the disease among the disparate ethnicities [12, 177].

One recent area of exploration is the involvement of DNA methylation and miRNA regulation. Epigenetic alterations are potentially reversible, and this possibility will facilitate the development of biomarkers and therapeutics in the prevailing disparities between AA and EA patients in HCC initiation and development. The identification and functional validation of race-specific methylation hotspots and miRNAs can be used to understand the mechanisms of disparities in HCC. This can be done by first identifying DNA methylation sites and miRNAs with statistically significant changes between HCC cases and cirrhotic or normal controls in a race-specific manner. Then, network-based methods and hierarchical integrative models can be used to integrate epigenomic data with transcriptomic, proteomic, glycoproteomic, and metabolomic data acquired from the same cirrhotic and HCC participants to select methylation hotspots and miRNAs relevant for understanding the mechanisms of disparities in HCC [177]. The selected candidates can then be validated by independent methods using frozen and formalin-fixed, paraffin-embedded (FFPE) liver tissues collected from patients with HCC and liver cirrhosis. Finally, functional validation of race-specific epigenetic modifications discovered in this type of high-throughput study can be performed through *in vitro* experiments using established cell lines derived from racially diverse populations. These cell cultures may present unique opportunities for targeted functional validation of epigenetic modifications and the downstream consequences.

In addition to exploring the external environment and how it influences HCC disease status, it is also necessary to explore the intestinal environment of different ethnicities. Experimental data from the obesity epidemic have revealed that the composition and products of the gut microbiome, which is altered with obesity and/or a high fat diet, are carcinogenic to the liver [187, 188]. Studies suggest that there are ethnic differences in microbial composition in a cirrhotic population at elevated risk for HCC as a result of metabolites, which can differentiate cirrhotic with HCC from those without HCC. Therefore, a case-control study can be designed to examine the contributions of race/ethnicity, fecal microbiome, fecal metabolome, and host factors (e.g., specific dietary factors and markers of body and liver fat composition) to NAFLD-related HCC. All in all, a multiethnic study of NAFLD and HCC that encompasses all racial/ethnic groups is needed to lay the groundwork for the elucidation of factors that account for health disparities across these populations. The prevalence of NAFLD is reported to be highest among Hispanics and Caucasians as mentioned above. However, NASH was the leading cause of waitlist LT registration in 2016 among Asian, Hispanic, and non-Hispanic white females, whereas HCV is still the leading cause in AA females [189].

As for gender differences in NAFLD or NASH, there are uncertainties including the role of IR in the influence of gender on NAFLD. Ruhl et al. reported that NAFLD is about 2.7 times more prevalent in men than in women [190]. One reasonable explanation for this reported gender difference in NAFLD is due to the higher waist-to-hip circumference (WHR) ratio in men [96]. Pan et al. further state that WHR is associated with visceral adipose tissue (VAT), which is correlated with both peripheral and hepatic IR. Similarly, in the Dallas Heart Study, European-American (EA) men had an approximately twofold higher prevalence of hepatic steatosis than EA women. This gender disparity has been blamed on alcohol use, sex hormones or lifestyle behaviors, and no differences in body weight or insulin sensitivity [96].

The ethnic distribution among NAFLD-/NASH-related HCC patients has yet to be defined [191]. If the increase in the number of ethnic groups waitlisted for LT from 2004 to 2016 is a good indicator of the rise in NASH-HCC, then it could be inferred from a recent retrospective study that Asian females had an 854% change in NASH waitlist registration, while Asian males had a 552% change [189]. The increase in African-American waitlist population was much less compared to the other ethnic groups. In contrast, the Hispanic females had a 3010% change in the rate of waitlist registration for NASH with HCC, while non-Hispanic white females had a 1992% change [189].

NASH-related HCC patients are primarily male even though gender is not a proven statistical risk factor in the progression of NASH to HCC. However, NASH is currently the second leading cause for LT waitlist in females, whereas in men, alcoholic liver disease (ALD) continues to be the leading cause [189]. Although old data of 698 patients from biopsy-proven NASH show that NASH patients are more likely to be female than male possibly reflecting a higher disease burden rate in women [192], it is likely that both gender and racial ethnic differences in NAFLD and NASH are attributed to interaction among genetic, environmental, and lifestyle behaviors.

5. Medical therapy for NAFLD and HCC

The biological heterogeneities of NAFLD and HCC create predicaments in deciphering the key mechanisms of development and progression from NAFLD to ESLD. Although progress is being made in understanding the molecular underpinnings of chronic liver disease and its various offshoots, there are still formidable challenges in providing effective treatment regimens. Aside from a few prophylactic agents that have shown promise in the prevention and treatment of steatohepatitis and fibrosis, there is no treatment consensus due to scarcity of data [140]. Wholesome lifestyle and behavioral changes that include regular physical activity, low caloric intake, and weight loss are the main bulwarks against NAFLD, which may progress to HCC with or without cirrhosis. However, the extent to which these modifications are effective to prevent the development of HCC is unclear. There is currently no effective chemoprevention to decrease the incidence of HCC except using nucleoside analogs to reduce viral replication for those infected with HBV [193] and direct-acting antivirals (DAAs) for those infected with HCV [194], the latter demonstrating very high cure rates but also raising concerns about the recurrence or development of HCC after the achievement of a sustained virological response [195]. Obeticholic acid (OCA), a selective agonist of the Farnesoid X receptors, was touted to be a promising pharmacological drug for the management of NAFLD. However, its low efficacy and specificity have dampened enthusiasm for its practical use. Also, the drug pioglitazone has no long-term impact on NASH. This entails a pressing need to develop more effective and safe agents for NAFLD and HCC. Several other experimental studies suggest a direct role for vitamin D in modulating liver fibrosis and inflammation by enhancing hepatic response to insulin via binding to vitamin D receptor on liver cells [196–198]. Vitamin E and carotenoids are also shown to decrease plasma levels of patients with NASH [199], whereas dietary antioxidants such as vitamin C and coenzyme Q12, trace minerals such as selenium, anticholesterol medications such as statins, antidiabetic drugs such as metformin, and methyl radical donors such as S-adenosylmethionine have all been touted as potential prophylactic agents [169, 200–202].

6. Key findings, future trends, and unmet needs

Hepatic steatosis is associated with many other morbidities. Therefore, dissecting the myriad causative agents including genetic, hormonal, or environmental factors underlying the pathogenicity of simple hepatic steatosis must be a priority to avoid the maze of complications that may arise during the development of NAFLD and its progression to HCC. The key findings are:

- Global prevalence of NAFLD is at 24% but is rising to greater than 30%; highest rates to lowest rates are found in South America, Middle East, Asia, United States, and Europe.

- The large volume of patients sets NAFLD apart from other liver diseases; thus, clinical care must focus on discerning highest risk of progressive liver disease.

- Overweight in childhood and adolescence is associated with the risk of NAFLD later in life and increases liver-related morbidity and/or mortality.

- NAFLD patients have an elevated risk of liver-related morbidity/mortality and metabolic comorbidities, which place a strain on healthcare systems.

- NAFLD warrants that primary-care physicians, specialists, and health policymakers stress prevention of excessive weight gain during childhood.

- Bariatric surgery may be an alternative option to committed weight loss.

- Older age, being male, and HA are independent risk factors for NAFLD/NASH.

- NAFLD is linked with higher BMI, higher HTN, and lower physical activity.

- MetS as currently defined is not a good predictor of NAFLD in non-Hispanic blacks (NHB); because in contrast to others, TG level is normal in this group.

- Proton magnetic resonance spectroscopy is currently the best proven alternative tool to biopsy for accurate diagnosis of NAFLD.

- Treatment options require more robust studies on etiology of NAFLD.

- There is no proven medical therapy for NASH.

- Most effective therapeutic strategies include lifestyle changes including diet, exercise, modifying metabolic risk factors, early screening, and intervention.

- Certain genes may be associated with disparities in lipid metabolism.

- Alternative noninvasive markers of NASH may now be available even though there are no proven biomarkers for various stages of the NAFLD spectrum.
- Discovery of new biomolecules during clinical trials and metabolomics studies is crucial for understanding NAFLD/NASH initiation and progression.
- Patients with NASH have a worse prognosis and must be included in clinical trials of new treatments.
- The biological heterogeneity of HCC makes it difficult to assess the key mechanisms of cancer development and thus implement effective therapies.
- Certain genes have been identified to be associated with progression to HCC.

Acknowledgements

This work was supported by the National Institutes of Health (NIH) Grant U01CA185188.

Conflicts of interest

The author has no conflict of interest.

Abbreviations

AA	African-American
AF	advanced fibrosis
ALT	alanine aminotransferase
AST	aspartate aminotransferase
BMI	body mass index
CDC	Centers for Disease Control and Prevention
DAA	direct-acting antiviral
EA	European-American
ESLD	end-stage liver disease
HA	Hispanic-American
HCC	hepatocellular carcinoma
HDL	high-density lipoprotein
HTN	hypertension
IR	insulin resistance
LT	liver transplantation
MetS	metabolic syndrome
NAFL	nonalcoholic fatty liver
NAFLD	nonalcoholic fatty liver disease
NASH	nonalcoholic steatohepatitis
NFS	NAFLD fibrosis score
NAS	NAFLD activity score
NHANES	National Health and Nutrition Examination Survey
NFS	NAFLD fibrosis score
T2DM	type 2 diabetes mellitus
TG	triglyceride
TCGA	the cancer genome atlas

Author details

Zaki A. Sherif
Department of Biochemistry and Molecular Biology, Howard University College of Medicine, Washington, DC, USA

*Address all correspondence to: zaki.sherif@howard.edu

IntechOpen

© 2019 The Author(s). Licensee IntechOpen. This chapter is distributed under the terms of the Creative Commons Attribution License (http://creativecommons.org/licenses/by/3.0), which permits unrestricted use, distribution, and reproduction in any medium, provided the original work is properly cited.

References

[1] Lear SA, Humphries KH, Kohli S, Birmingham CL. The use of BMI and waist circumference as surrogates of body fat differs by ethnicity. Obesity. 2007;**15**:2817-2824

[2] Dongiovanni P, Anstee QM, Valenti L. Genetic predisposition in NAFLD and NASH: Impact on severity of liver disease and response to treatment. Current Pharmaceutical Design. 2013;**19**:5219-5238

[3] Marengo A, Rosso C, Bugianesi E. Liver cancer: Connections with obesity, fatty liver, and cirrhosis. Annual Review of Medicine. 2016;**67**:103-117

[4] Estes C, Razavi H, Loomba R, Younossi Z, Sanyal AJ. Modeling the epidemic of nonalcoholic fatty liver disease demonstrates an exponential increase in burden of disease. Hepatology. 2018;**67**:123-133

[5] Bedossa P, Poitou C, Veyrie N, et al. Histopathological algorithm and scoring system for evaluation of liver lesions in morbidly obese patients. Hepatology. 2012;**56**:1751-1759

[6] Kleiner DE, Brunt EM, Van Natta M, et al. Design and validation of a histological scoring system for nonalcoholic fatty liver disease. Hepatology. 2005;**41**:1313-1321

[7] Ballestri S, Nascimbeni F, Baldelli E, Marrazzo A, Romagnoli D, Lonardo A. NAFLD as a sexual dimorphic disease: Role of gender and reproductive status in the development and progression of nonalcoholic fatty liver disease and inherent cardiovascular risk. Advances in Therapy. 2017;**34**:1291-1326

[8] Ogden CL, Carroll MD, Lawman HG, et al. Trends in obesity prevalence among children and adolescents in the United States, 1988-1994 through 2013-2014. Journal of the American Medical Association. 2016;**315**:2292-2299

[9] Flegal KM, Kruszon-Moran D, Carroll MD, Fryar CD, Ogden CL. Trends in obesity among adults in the United States, 2005 to 2014. Journal of the American Medical Association. 2016;**315**:2284-2291

[10] Malik SM, Ahmad J. Outcomes of liver transplantation in patients with cirrhosis due to nonalcoholic steatohepatitis versus patients with cirrhosis due to alcoholic liver disease. Liver Transplantation. 2010;**16**:533

[11] Farrell GC, Larter CZ. Nonalcoholic fatty liver disease: From steatosis to cirrhosis. Hepatology. 2006;**43**:S99-S112

[12] Benedict M, Zhang X. Non-alcoholic fatty liver disease: An expanded review. World Journal of Hepatology. 2017;**9**:715-732

[13] Loomba R, Sanyal AJ. The global NAFLD epidemic. Nature Reviews Gastroenterology & Hepatology. 2013;**10**:686-690

[14] Sayiner M, Koenig A, Henry L, Younossi ZM. Epidemiology of nonalcoholic fatty liver disease and nonalcoholic steatohepatitis in the United States and the rest of the world. Clinics in Liver Disease. 2016;**20**:205-214

[15] Ruhl CE, Everhart JE. Fatty liver indices in the multiethnic United States National Health and Nutrition Examination Survey. Alimentary Pharmacology & Therapeutics. 2015;**41**:65-76

[16] Younossi Z, Anstee QM, Marietti M, et al. Global burden of NAFLD and NASH: Trends, predictions, risk factors and prevention. Nature Reviews Gastroenterology & Hepatology. 2018;**15**:11-20

[17] GBD 2016 Alcohol Collaborators. Alcohol use and burden for 195 countries and territories, 1990-2016:

A systematic analysis for the global burden of disease study 2016. Lancet. 2018;**392**:1015-1035

[18] Hajifathalian K, Torabi Sagvand B, McCullough AJ. Effect of alcohol consumption on survival in nonalcoholic fatty liver disease: A National Prospective Cohort Study. Hepatology. 2018. DOI: 10.1002/hep.30226

[19] Younossi ZM, Stepanova M, Ong J, et al. Effects of alcohol consumption and metabolic syndrome on mortality in patients with non-alcoholic and alcohol-related fatty liver disease. Clinical Gastroenterology and Hepatology. 2018;**17**:1625-1633

[20] Wood AM, Kaptoge S, Butterworth AS, et al. Risk thresholds for alcohol consumption: Combined analysis of individual-participant data for 599 912 current drinkers in 83 prospective studies. Lancet. 2018;**391**:1513-1523

[21] Mantovani A. Time to revise the definition of NAFLD: A purist vision. Digestive and Liver Disease. 2019;**51**;457-458

[22] Gao X, Fan JG, Study Group of Liver and Metabolism, Chinese Society of Endocrinology. Diagnosis and management of non-alcoholic fatty liver disease and related metabolic disorders: Consensus statement from the Study Group of Liver and Metabolism, Chinese Society of Endocrinology. Journal of Diabetes. 2013;**5**:406-415

[23] Chalasani N, Younossi Z, Lavine JE, et al. The diagnosis and management of non-alcoholic fatty liver disease: Practice guideline by the American Gastroenterological Association, American Association for the Study of Liver Diseases, and American College of Gastroenterology. Gastroenterology. 2012;**142**:1592-1609

[24] Cobbold JF, Anstee QM, Thomas HC. Investigating mildly abnormal serum aminotransferase values. British Medical Journal. 2010;**341**:c4039

[25] Farrell GC, Chitturi S, Lau GK, Sollano JD. Asia-Pacific working party on NAFLD. Guidelines for the assessment and management of non-alcoholic fatty liver disease in the Asia-Pacific region: Executive summary. Journal of Gastroenterology and Hepatology. 2007;**22**:775-777

[26] Pais R, Rusu E, Zilisteanu D, et al. Prevalence of steatosis and insulin resistance in patients with chronic hepatitis B compared with chronic hepatitis C and non-alcoholic fatty liver disease. European Journal of Internal Medicine. 2015;**26**:30-36

[27] Bellentani S, Scaglioni F, Marino M, Bedogni G. Epidemiology of non-alcoholic fatty liver disease. Digestive Diseases. 2010;**28**:155-161

[28] Sattar N, Forrest E, Preiss D. Non-alcoholic fatty liver disease. British Medical Journal. 2014;**349**:g4596

[29] Sakhuja P. Pathology of alcoholic liver disease, can it be differentiated from nonalcoholic steatohepatitis? World Journal of Gastroenterology. 2014;**20**:16474-16479

[30] Neuman MG, French SW, French BA, et al. Alcoholic and non-alcoholic steatohepatitis. Experimental and Molecular Pathology. 2014;**97**:492-510

[31] Dumitrascu DL, Neuman MG. Non-alcoholic fatty liver disease: An update on diagnosis. Clujul Medical. 2018;**91**:147-150

[32] Powell EE, Jonsson JR, Clouston AD. Steatosis: Co-factor in other liver diseases. Hepatology. 2005;**42**:5-13

[33] Angulo P, Kleiner DE, Dam-Larsen S, et al. Liver fibrosis, but no other histologic features, is associated

with long-term outcomes of patients with nonalcoholic fatty liver disease. Gastroenterology. 2015;**149**:389-397.e10

[34] Adams LA, Lymp JF, St Sauver J, et al. The natural history of nonalcoholic fatty liver disease: A population-based cohort study. Gastroenterology. 2005;**129**:113-121

[35] Ekstedt M, Franzen LE, Mathiesen UL, et al. Long-term follow-up of patients with NAFLD and elevated liver enzymes. Hepatology. 2006;**44**:865-873

[36] Ekstedt M, Hagstrom H, Nasr P, et al. Fibrosis stage is the strongest predictor for disease-specific mortality in NAFLD after up to 33 years of follow-up. Hepatology. 2015;**61**:1547-1554

[37] Matteoni CA, Younossi ZM, Gramlich T, Boparai N, Liu YC, McCullough AJ. Nonalcoholic fatty liver disease: A spectrum of clinical and pathological severity. Gastroenterology. 1999;**116**:1413-1419

[38] Teli MR, James OF, Burt AD, Bennett MK, Day CP. The natural history of nonalcoholic fatty liver: A follow-up study. Hepatology. 1995;**22**:1714-1719

[39] Dyson JK, Anstee QM, McPherson S. Non-alcoholic fatty liver disease: A practical approach to diagnosis and staging. Frontline Gastroenterology. 2014;**5**:211-218

[40] Browning JD, Szczepaniak LS, Dobbins R, et al. Prevalence of hepatic steatosis in an urban population in the United States: Impact of ethnicity. Hepatology. 2004;**40**:1387-1395

[41] Wong VW, Chu WC, Wong GL, et al. Prevalence of non-alcoholic fatty liver disease and advanced fibrosis in Hong Kong Chinese: A population study using proton-magnetic resonance spectroscopy and transient elastography. Gut. 2012;**61**:409-415

[42] Sanyal AJ, Banas C, Sargeant C, et al. Similarities and differences in outcomes of cirrhosis due to nonalcoholic steatohepatitis and hepatitis C. Hepatology. 2006;**43**:682-689

[43] Lindvig KP, Teisner AS, Kjeldsen J, et al. Allocation of patients with liver cirrhosis and organ failure to intensive care: Systematic review and a proposal for clinical practice. World Journal of Gastroenterology. 2015;**21**:8964-8973

[44] Turchinovich A, Baranova A, Drapkina O, Tonevitsky A. Cell-free circulating nucleic acids as early biomarkers for NAFLD and NAFLD-associated disorders. Frontiers in Physiology. 2018;**9**:1256

[45] Neuschwander-Tetri BA, Caldwell SH. Nonalcoholic steatohepatitis: Summary of an AASLD single topic conference. Hepatology. 2003;**37**:1202-1219

[46] American Gastroenterological Association. American Gastro-enterological Association medical position statement: Nonalcoholic fatty liver disease. Gastroenterology. 2002;**123**:1702-1704

[47] Dixon JB, Bhathal PS, O'Brien PE. Nonalcoholic fatty liver disease: Predictors of nonalcoholic steatohepatitis and liver fibrosis in the severely obese. Gastroenterology. 2001;**121**:91-100

[48] Strauss S, Gavish E, Gottlieb P, Katsnelson L. Interobserver and intraobserver variability in the sonographic assessment of fatty liver. AJR. American Journal of Roentgenology. 2007;**189**:W320-W323

[49] Saadeh S, Younossi ZM, Remer EM, et al. The utility of radiological imaging in nonalcoholic fatty liver disease. Gastroenterology. 2002;**123**:745-750

[50] Schwenzer NF, Springer F, Schraml C, Stefan N, Machann J, Schick F. Non-invasive assessment and quantification of liver steatosis by ultrasound, computed tomography and magnetic resonance. Journal of Hepatology. 2009;**51**:433-445

[51] McPherson S, Jonsson JR, Cowin GJ, et al. Magnetic resonance imaging and spectroscopy accurately estimate the severity of steatosis provided the stage of fibrosis is considered. Journal of Hepatology. 2009;**51**:389-397

[52] Li Q, Dhyani M, Grajo JR, Sirlin C, Samir AE. Current status of imaging in nonalcoholic fatty liver disease. World Journal of Hepatology. 2018;**10**:530-542

[53] Lee SS, Park SH. Radiologic evaluation of nonalcoholic fatty liver disease. World Journal of Gastroenterology. 2014;**20**:7392-7402

[54] Wang Y, Fan Q, Wang T, Wen J, Wang H, Zhang T. Controlled attenuation parameter for assessment of hepatic steatosis grades: A diagnostic meta-analysis. International Journal of Clinical and Experimental Medicine. 2015;**8**:17654-17663

[55] Streba LA, Vere CC, Rogoveanu I, Streba CT. Nonalcoholic fatty liver disease, metabolic risk factors, and hepatocellular carcinoma: An open question. World Journal of Gastroenterology. 2015;**21**:4103-4110

[56] Bril F, Cusi K. Management of nonalcoholic fatty liver disease in patients with type 2 diabetes: A call to action. Diabetes Care. 2017;**40**:419-430

[57] Mofrad P, Contos MJ, Haque M, et al. Clinical and histologic spectrum of nonalcoholic fatty liver disease associated with normal ALT values. Hepatology. 2003;**37**:1286-1292

[58] Yano E, Tagawa K, Yamaoka K, Mori M. Test validity of periodic liver function tests in a population of Japanese male bank employees. Journal of Clinical Epidemiology. 2001;**54**:945-951

[59] Martin-Rodriguez JL, Gonzalez-Cantero J, Gonzalez-Cantero A, Arrebola JP, Gonzalez-Calvin JL. Diagnostic accuracy of serum alanine aminotransferase as biomarker for nonalcoholic fatty liver disease and insulin resistance in healthy subjects, using 3T MR spectroscopy. Medicine. 2017;**96**:e6770

[60] Oh RC, Hustead TR, Ali SM, Pantsari MW. Mildly elevated liver transaminase levels: Causes and evaluation. American Family Physician. 2017;**96**:709-715

[61] Sherif ZA, Saeed A, Ghavimi S, et al. Global epidemiology of nonalcoholic fatty liver disease and perspectives on US minority populations. Digestive Diseases and Sciences. 2016;**61**:1214-1225

[62] Feldstein AE, Canbay A, Angulo P, et al. Hepatocyte apoptosis and fas expression are prominent features of human nonalcoholic steatohepatitis. Gastroenterology. 2003;**125**:437-443

[63] Bantel H, Ruck P, Gregor M, Schulze-Osthoff K. Detection of elevated caspase activation and early apoptosis in liver diseases. European Journal of Cell Biology. 2001;**80**:230-239

[64] Feldstein AE, Wieckowska A, Lopez AR, Liu YC, Zein NN, McCullough AJ. Cytokeratin-18 fragment levels as noninvasive biomarkers for nonalcoholic steatohepatitis: A multicenter validation study. Hepatology. 2009;**50**:1072-1078

[65] Younossi ZM, Koenig AB, Abdelatif D, Fazel Y, Henry L, Wymer M. Global epidemiology of nonalcoholic fatty liver disease-meta-analytic assessment of

prevalence, incidence, and outcomes. Hepatology. 2016;**64**:73-84

[66] Merriman RB, Ferrell LD, Patti MG, et al. Correlation of paired liver biopsies in morbidly obese patients with suspected nonalcoholic fatty liver disease. Hepatology. 2006;**44**:874-880

[67] Bhatt HB, Smith RJ. Fatty liver disease in diabetes mellitus. Hepatobiliary Surgery and Nutrition. 2015;**4**:101-108

[68] Pinto RB, Schneider AC, da Silveira TR. Cirrhosis in children and adolescents: An overview. World Journal of Hepatology. 2015;7:392-405

[69] Anstee QM, McPherson S, Day CP. How big a problem is non-alcoholic fatty liver disease? British Medical Journal. 2011;**343**:d3897

[70] Sandrin L, Fourquet B, Hasquenoph JM, et al. Transient elastography: A new noninvasive method for assessment of hepatic fibrosis. Ultrasound in Medicine & Biology. 2003;**29**:1705-1713

[71] Dahl JJ, Pinton GF, Palmeri ML, Agrawal V, Nightingale KR, Trahey GE. A parallel tracking method for acoustic radiation force impulse imaging. IEEE Transactions on Ultrasonics, Ferroelectrics, and Frequency Control. 2007;**54**:301-312

[72] Gregg EW, Boyle JP, Thompson TJ, Barker LE, Albright AL, Williamson DF. Modeling the impact of prevention policies on future diabetes prevalence in the United States: 2010-2030. Population Health Metrics. 2013;**11**:18

[73] Koehler EM, Plompen EP, Schouten JN, et al. Presence of diabetes mellitus and steatosis is associated with liver stiffness in a general population: The Rotterdam study. Hepatology. 2016;**63**:138-147

[74] Rosenberg WM, Voelker M, Thiel R, et al. Serum markers detect the presence of liver fibrosis: A cohort study. Gastroenterology. 2004;**127**:1704-1713

[75] Rotman Y, Koh C, Zmuda JM, Kleiner DE, Liang TJ, NASH CRN. The association of genetic variability in patatin-like phospholipase domain-containing protein 3 (PNPLA3) with histological severity of nonalcoholic fatty liver disease. Hepatology. 2010;**52**:894-903

[76] Anstee QM, Targher G, Day CP. Progression of NAFLD to diabetes mellitus, cardiovascular disease or cirrhosis. Nature Reviews Gastroenterology & Hepatology. 2013;**10**:330-344

[77] Demir M, Lang S, Steffen HM. Nonalcoholic fatty liver disease: Current status and future directions. Journal of Digestive Diseases. 2015;**16**:541-557

[78] Grundy SM. Obesity, metabolic syndrome, and cardiovascular disease. The Journal of Clinical Endocrinology and Metabolism. 2004;**89**:2595-2600

[79] Grundy SM, Cleeman JI, Daniels SR, et al. Diagnosis and management of the metabolic syndrome: An American Heart Association/National Heart, Lung, and Blood Institute scientific statement: Executive summary. Critical Pathways in Cardiology. 2005;**4**:198-203

[80] Hassan MM, Curley SA, Li D, et al. Association of diabetes duration and diabetes treatment with the risk of hepatocellular carcinoma. Cancer. 2010;**116**:1938-1946

[81] American Diabetes Association. Diagnosis and classification of diabetes mellitus. Diabetes Care. 2009;**32** (Suppl 1):S62-S67

[82] Ballestri S, Zona S, Targher G, et al. Nonalcoholic fatty liver disease is associated with an almost twofold increased risk of incident type 2 diabetes and metabolic syndrome. Evidence from

a systematic review and meta-analysis. Journal of Gastroenterology and Hepatology. 2016;**31**:936-944

[83] Ahmed MH, Abu EO, Byrne CD. Non-alcoholic fatty liver disease (NAFLD): New challenge for general practitioners and important burden for health authorities? Primary Care Diabetes. 2010;**4**:129-137

[84] Portillo-Sanchez P, Bril F, Maximos M, et al. High prevalence of nonalcoholic fatty liver disease in patients with type 2 diabetes mellitus and normal plasma aminotransferase levels. The Journal of Clinical Endocrinology and Metabolism. 2015;**100**:2231-2238

[85] Adams LA, Waters OR, Knuiman MW, Elliott RR, Olynyk JK. NAFLD as a risk factor for the development of diabetes and the metabolic syndrome: An eleven-year follow-up study. The American Journal of Gastroenterology. 2009;**104**:861-867

[86] McCullough AJ. Epidemiology of the metabolic syndrome in the USA. Journal of Digestive Diseases. 2011;**12**:333-340

[87] Ruan H, Lodish HF. Insulin resistance in adipose tissue: Direct and indirect effects of tumor necrosis factor-alpha. Cytokine & Growth Factor Reviews. 2003;**14**:447-455

[88] Uysal KT, Wiesbrock SM, Marino MW, Hotamisligil GS. Protection from obesity-induced insulin resistance in mice lacking TNF-alpha function. Nature. 1997;**389**:610-614

[89] Angulo P, Keach JC, Batts KP, Lindor KD. Independent predictors of liver fibrosis in patients with nonalcoholic steatohepatitis. Hepatology. 1999;**30**:1356-1362

[90] Friedenberg F, Pungpapong S, Zaeri N, Braitman LE. The impact of diabetes and obesity on liver histology in patients with hepatitis C. Diabetes, Obesity & Metabolism. 2003;**5**:150-155

[91] Adinolfi LE, Gambardella M, Andreana A, Tripodi MF, Utili R, Ruggiero G. Steatosis accelerates the progression of liver damage of chronic hepatitis C patients and correlates with specific HCV genotype and visceral obesity. Hepatology. 2001;**33**:1358-1364

[92] Pekow JR, Bhan AK, Zheng H, Chung RT. Hepatic steatosis is associated with increased frequency of hepatocellular carcinoma in patients with hepatitis C-related cirrhosis. Cancer. 2007;**109**:2490-2496

[93] Leandro G, Mangia A, Hui J, et al. Relationship between steatosis, inflammation, and fibrosis in chronic hepatitis C: A meta-analysis of individual patient data. Gastroenterology. 2006;**130**:1636-1642

[94] Afsari A, Lee E, Shokrani B, et al. Clinical and pathological risk factors associated with liver fibrosis and steatosis in African-Americans with chronic hepatitis C. Digestive Diseases and Sciences. 2017;**62**:2159-2165

[95] Bambha K, Belt P, Abraham M, et al. Ethnicity and nonalcoholic fatty liver disease. Hepatology. 2012;**55**:769-780

[96] Pan JJ, Fallon MB. Gender and racial differences in nonalcoholic fatty liver disease. World Journal of Hepatology. 2014;**6**:274-283

[97] Sliz E, Sebert S, Wurtz P, et al. NAFLD risk alleles in PNPLA3, TM6SF2, GCKR and LYPLAL1 show divergent metabolic effects. Human Molecular Genetics. 2018;**27**:2214-2223

[98] Yang Z, Wen J, Tao X, et al. Genetic variation in the GCKR gene is associated with non-alcoholic fatty liver disease in Chinese people. Molecular Biology Reports. 2011;**38**:1145-1150

[99] Bruschi FV, Tardelli M, Claudel T, Trauner M. PNPLA3 expression and its impact on the liver: Current perspectives. Hepatic Medicine : Evidence And Research. 2017;**9**:55-66

[100] Palmer ND, Musani SK, Yerges-Armstrong LM, et al. Characterization of European ancestry nonalcoholic fatty liver disease-associated variants in individuals of African and Hispanic descent. Hepatology. 2013;**58**:966-975

[101] Romeo S, Huang-Doran I, Baroni MG, Kotronen A. Unravelling the pathogenesis of fatty liver disease: Patatin-like phospholipase domain-containing 3 protein. Current Opinion in Lipidology. 2010;**21**:247-252

[102] Romeo S, Kozlitina J, Xing C, et al. Genetic variation in PNPLA3 confers susceptibility to nonalcoholic fatty liver disease. Nature Genetics. 2008;**40**:1461-1465

[103] Singal AG, Manjunath H, Yopp AC, et al. The effect of PNPLA3 on fibrosis progression and development of hepatocellular carcinoma: A meta-analysis. The American Journal of Gastroenterology. 2014;**109**:325-334

[104] Kozlitina J, Smagris E, Stender S, et al. Exome-wide association study identifies a TM6SF2 variant that confers susceptibility to nonalcoholic fatty liver disease. Nature Genetics. 2014;**46**:352-356

[105] Britton LJ, Subramaniam VN, Crawford DH. Iron and non-alcoholic fatty liver disease. World Journal of Gastroenterology. 2016;**22**:8112-8122

[106] Miyake T, Kumagi T, Furukawa S, et al. Non-alcoholic fatty liver disease: Factors associated with its presence and onset. Journal of Gastroenterology and Hepatology. 2013;**28**(Suppl 4):71-78

[107] Zhao F. Dysregulated epigenetic modifications in the pathogenesis of NAFLD-HCC. Advances in Experimental Medicine and Biology. 2018;**1061**:79-93

[108] de Mello VD, Matte A, Perfilyev A, et al. Human liver epigenetic alterations in non-alcoholic steatohepatitis are related to insulin action. Epigenetics. 2017;**12**:287-295

[109] Cordero P, Campion J, Milagro FI, Martinez JA. Transcriptomic and epigenetic changes in early liver steatosis associated to obesity: Effect of dietary methyl donor supplementation. Molecular Genetics and Metabolism. 2013;**110**:388-395

[110] Mouralidarane A, Soeda J, Sugden D, et al. Maternal obesity programs offspring non-alcoholic fatty liver disease through disruption of 24-h rhythms in mice. International Journal of Obesity. 2015;**39**:1339-1348

[111] Oben JA, Mouralidarane A, Samuelsson AM, et al. Maternal obesity during pregnancy and lactation programs the development of offspring non-alcoholic fatty liver disease in mice. Journal of Hepatology. 2010;**52**:913-920

[112] Aron-Wisnewsky J, Gaborit B, Dutour A, Clement K. Gut microbiota and non-alcoholic fatty liver disease: New insights. Clinical Microbiology and Infection. 2013;**19**:338-348

[113] Henao-Mejia J, Elinav E, Jin C, et al. Inflammasome-mediated dysbiosis regulates progression of NAFLD and obesity. Nature. 2012;**482**:179-185

[114] Gerhard GS, Malenica I, Llaci L, et al. Differentially methylated loci in NAFLD cirrhosis are associated with key signaling pathways. Clinical Epigenetics. 2018;**10**:93

[115] Garcia-Monzon C, Petrov PD, Rey E, et al. Angiopoietin-like protein 8 is

a novel vitamin D receptor target gene involved in non-alcoholic fatty liver pathogenesis. The American Journal of Pathology. 2018;**188**:2800-2810

[116] Blond E, Disse E, Cuerq C, et al. EASL-EASD-EASO clinical practice guidelines for the management of non-alcoholic fatty liver disease in severely obese people: Do they lead to over-referral? Diabetologia. 2017;**60**:1218-1222

[117] Nasr P, Ignatova S, Kechagias S, Ekstedt M. Natural history of nonalcoholic fatty liver disease: A prospective follow-up study with serial biopsies. Hepatology Communications. 2017;**2**:199-210

[118] Lindenmeyer CC, McCullough AJ. The natural history of nonalcoholic fatty liver disease-an evolving view. Clinics in Liver Disease. 2018;**22**:11-21

[119] Guerrero R, Vega GL, Grundy SM, Browning JD. Ethnic differences in hepatic steatosis: An insulin resistance paradox? Hepatology. 2009;**49**:791-801

[120] Angulo P. Nonalcoholic fatty liver disease. The New England Journal of Medicine. 2002;**346**:1221-1231

[121] Rinella ME. Nonalcoholic fatty liver disease: A systematic review. Journal of the American Medical Association. 2015;**313**:2263-2273

[122] Lazo M, Hernaez R, Eberhardt MS, et al. Prevalence of nonalcoholic fatty liver disease in the United States: The third National Health and Nutrition Examination Survey, 1988-1994. American Journal of Epidemiology. 2013;**178**:38-45

[123] Younossi ZM, Otgonsuren M, Henry L, et al. Association of nonalcoholic fatty liver disease (NAFLD) with hepatocellular carcinoma (HCC) in the United States from 2004 to 2009. Hepatology. 2015;**62**:1723-1730

[124] Pais R, Barritt AS 4th, Calmus Y, et al. NAFLD and liver transplantation: Current burden and expected challenges. Journal of Hepatology. 2016;**65**:1245-1257

[125] White DL, Kanwal F, El-Serag HB. Association between nonalcoholic fatty liver disease and risk for hepatocellular cancer, based on systematic review. Clinical Gastroenterology and Hepatology. 2012;**10**:1342-1359.e2

[126] Starley BQ, Calcagno CJ, Harrison SA. Nonalcoholic fatty liver disease and hepatocellular carcinoma: A weighty connection. Hepatology. 2010;**51**:1820-1832

[127] Kawada N, Imanaka K, Kawaguchi T, et al. Hepatocellular carcinoma arising from non-cirrhotic nonalcoholic steatohepatitis. Journal of Gastroenterology. 2009;**44**:1190-1194

[128] Castera L, Friedrich-Rust M, Loomba R. Non-invasive assessment of liver disease in patients with NAFLD. Gastroenterology. 2019;**156**:1264-1281

[129] Papastergiou V, Tsochatzis E, Burroughs AK. Non-invasive assessment of liver fibrosis. Annals of Gastroenterology. 2012;**25**:218-231

[130] Angulo P, Hui JM, Marchesini G, et al. The NAFLD fibrosis score: A noninvasive system that identifies liver fibrosis in patients with NAFLD. Hepatology. 2007;**45**:846-854

[131] Matsushita N, Hassanein MT, Martinez-Clemente M, et al. Gender difference in NASH susceptibility: Roles of hepatocyte Ikkbeta and Sult1e1. PLoS One. 2017;**12**:e0181052. DOI: 10.1371/journal.pone.0181052

[132] Machado MV, Cortez-Pinto H. Non-invasive diagnosis of non-alcoholic fatty liver disease. A critical

appraisal. Journal of Hepatology. 2013;**58**:1007-1019

[133] Sookoian S, Castano GO, Burgueno AL, Gianotti TF, Rosselli MS, Pirola CJ. A nonsynonymous gene variant in the adiponutrin gene is associated with nonalcoholic fatty liver disease severity. Journal of Lipid Research. 2009;**50**:2111-2116

[134] Ouyang X, Cirillo P, Sautin Y, et al. Fructose consumption as a risk factor for non-alcoholic fatty liver disease. Journal of Hepatology. 2008;**48**:993-999

[135] Musso G, Gambino R, De Michieli F, et al. Dietary habits and their relations to insulin resistance and postprandial lipemia in nonalcoholic steatohepatitis. Hepatology. 2003;**37**:909-916

[136] Cortez-Pinto H, Jesus L, Barros H, Lopes C, Moura MC, Camilo ME. How different is the dietary pattern in non-alcoholic steatohepatitis patients? Clinical Nutrition. 2006;**25**:816-823

[137] Musso G, Cassader M, Olivetti C, Rosina F, Carbone G, Gambino R. Association of obstructive sleep apnoea with the presence and severity of non-alcoholic fatty liver disease. A systematic review and meta-analysis. Obesity Reviews. 2013;**14**:417-431

[138] Byrne CD, Olufadi R, Bruce KD, Cagampang FR, Ahmed MH. Metabolic disturbances in non-alcoholic fatty liver disease. Clinical Science. 2009;**116**:539-564

[139] Williams CD, Stengel J, Asike MI, et al. Prevalence of nonalcoholic fatty liver disease and nonalcoholic steatohepatitis among a largely middle-aged population utilizing ultrasound and liver biopsy: A prospective study. Gastroenterology. 2011;**140**:124-131

[140] Cholankeril G, Patel R, Khurana S, Satapathy SK. Hepatocellular carcinoma in non-alcoholic steatohepatitis: Current knowledge and implications for management. World Journal of Hepatology. 2017;**9**:533-543

[141] Torre LA, Bray F, Siegel RL, Ferlay J, Lortet-Tieulent J, Jemal A. Global cancer statistics, 2012. CA: A Cancer Journal for Clinicians. 2015;**65**:87-108

[142] El-Serag HB. Hepatocellular carcinoma. The New England Journal of Medicine. 2011;**365**:1118-1127

[143] Zucman-Rossi J, Villanueva A, Nault JC, Llovet JM. Genetic landscape and biomarkers of hepatocellular carcinoma. Gastroenterology. 2015;**149**:1226-1239.e4

[144] Llovet JM, Zucman-Rossi J, Pikarsky E, et al. Hepatocellular carcinoma. Nature Reviews Disease Primers. 2016;**2**:16018

[145] McGlynn KA, London WT. The global epidemiology of hepatocellular carcinoma: Present and future. Clinics in Liver Disease. 2011;**15**:223-243, vii-x

[146] Pittman ME, Brunt EM. Anatomic pathology of hepatocellular carcinoma: Histopathology using classic and new diagnostic tools. Clinics in Liver Disease. 2015;**19**:239-259

[147] Rastogi A. Changing role of histopathology in the diagnosis and management of hepatocellular carcinoma. World Journal of Gastroenterology. 2018;**24**:4000-4013

[148] Margini C, Dufour JF. The story of HCC in NAFLD: From epidemiology, across pathogenesis, to prevention and treatment. Liver International. 2016;**36**:317-324

[149] Michelotti GA, Machado MV, Diehl AM. NAFLD, NASH and liver cancer. Nature Reviews Gastroenterology & Hepatology. 2013;**10**:656-665

[150] Baffy G, Brunt EM, Caldwell SH. Hepatocellular carcinoma in non-alcoholic fatty liver disease: An emerging menace. Journal of Hepatology. 2012;**56**:1384-1391

[151] Marrero JA, Fontana RJ, Su GL, Conjeevaram HS, Emick DM, Lok AS. NAFLD may be a common underlying liver disease in patients with hepatocellular carcinoma in the United States. Hepatology. 2002;**36**:1349-1354

[152] Bugianesi E, Leone N, Vanni E, et al. Expanding the natural history of nonalcoholic steatohepatitis: From cryptogenic cirrhosis to hepatocellular carcinoma. Gastroenterology. 2002;**123**:134-140

[153] Singh AK, Kumar R, Pandey AK. Hepatocellular carcinoma: Causes, mechanism of progression and biomarkers. Current Chemical Genomics and Translational Medicine. 2018;**12**:9-26

[154] Jayachandran M. An updated portrait of pathogenesis, molecular markers and signaling pathways of hepatocellular carcinoma. Current Pharmaceutical Design. 2017;**23**:2356-2365

[155] Liu Y, Yang Z, Du F, et al. Molecular mechanisms of pathogenesis in hepatocellular carcinoma revealed by RNA-sequencing. Molecular Medicine Reports. 2017;**16**:6674-6682

[156] Chen J, Qian Z, Li F, Li J, Lu Y. Integrative analysis of microarray data to reveal regulation patterns in the pathogenesis of hepatocellular carcinoma. Gut and Liver. 2017;**11**:112-120

[157] Cancer Genome Atlas Research Network. Electronic address: wheeler@bcm.edu, Cancer Genome Atlas Research Network. Comprehensive and integrative genomic characterization of hepatocellular carcinoma. Cell. 2017;**169**:1327-1341.e23

[158] Huang MN, Yu W, Teoh WW, et al. Genome-scale mutational signatures of aflatoxin in cells, mice, and human tumors. Genome Research. 2017;**27**:1475-1486

[159] Tahmasebi Birgani M, Carloni V. Tumor microenvironment, a paradigm in hepatocellular carcinoma progression and therapy. International Journal of Molecular Sciences. 2017;**18**:pii.E405. DOI: 10.3390/ijms18020405

[160] Meng C, Shen X, Jiang W. Potential biomarkers of HCC based on gene expression and DNA methylation profiles. Oncology Letters. 2018;**16**:3183-3192

[161] De Mattia E, Cecchin E, Polesel J, et al. Genetic biomarkers for hepatocellular cancer risk in a caucasian population. World Journal of Gastroenterology. 2017;**23**:6674-6684

[162] Li B, Xu T, Liu C, et al. Liver-enriched genes are associated with the prognosis of patients with hepatocellular carcinoma. Scientific Reports. 2018;**8**:11197

[163] Xu J, Wu C, Che X, et al. Circulating microRNAs, miR-21, miR-122, and miR-223, in patients with hepatocellular carcinoma or chronic hepatitis. Molecular Carcinogenesis. 2011;**50**:136-142

[164] Wong CM, Tsang FH, Ng IO. Non-coding RNAs in hepatocellular carcinoma: Molecular functions and pathological implications. Nature Reviews Gastroenterology & Hepatology. 2018;**15**:137-151

[165] Rinella ME. Will the increased prevalence of nonalcoholic steatohepatitis (NASH) in the age of better hepatitis C virus therapy make NASH the deadlier disease? Hepatology. 2011;**54**:1118-1120

[166] Armstrong MJ, Houlihan DD, Bentham L, et al. Presence and severity

of non-alcoholic fatty liver disease in a large prospective primary care cohort. Journal of Hepatology. 2012;**56**:234-240

[167] Ofosu A, Ramai D, Reddy M. Non-alcoholic fatty liver disease: Controlling an emerging epidemic, challenges, and future directions. Annals of Gastroenterology. 2018;**31**:288-295

[168] Goldberg D, Ditah IC, Saeian K, et al. Changes in the prevalence of hepatitis C virus infection, nonalcoholic steatohepatitis, and alcoholic liver disease among patients with cirrhosis or liver failure on the waitlist for liver transplantation. Gastroenterology. 2017;**152**:1090-1099.e1

[169] Noureddin M, Rinella ME. Nonalcoholic fatty liver disease, diabetes, obesity, and hepatocellular carcinoma. Clinics in Liver Disease. 2015;**19**:361-379

[170] Wong RJ, Cheung R, Ahmed A. Nonalcoholic steatohepatitis is the most rapidly growing indication for liver transplantation in patients with hepatocellular carcinoma in the U.S. Hepatology. 2014;**59**:2188-2195

[171] Portillo Sanchez P, Bril F, Maximos M, et al. High prevalence of nonalcoholic fatty liver disease in patients with type 2 diabetes mellitus and normal plasma aminotransferase levels. The Journal of Clinical Endocrinology and Metabolism. 2014;**100**:2231-2238. DOI: 10.1210/jc.2014-2739

[172] Parikh ND, Marrero WJ, Wang J, et al. Projected increase in obesity and non-alcoholic-steatohepatitis-related liver transplantation waitlist additions in the United States. Hepatology. 2017. DOI: 10.1002/hep.29473

[173] Schneider AL, Lazo M, Selvin E, Clark JM. Racial differences in nonalcoholic fatty liver disease in the U.S. population. Obesity. 2014;**22**:292-299

[174] Weston SR, Leyden W, Murphy R, et al. Racial and ethnic distribution of nonalcoholic fatty liver in persons with newly diagnosed chronic liver disease. Hepatology. 2005;**41**:372-379

[175] Caldwell SH, Harris DM, Patrie JT, Hespenheide EE. Is NASH underdiagnosed among African Americans? The American Journal of Gastroenterology. 2002;**97**:1496-1500

[176] Morgan C, Mallett R, Hutchinson G, et al. Pathways to care and ethnicity. 2: Source of referral and help-seeking. Report from the AESOP study. The British Journal of Psychiatry. 2005;**186**:290-296

[177] Di Poto C, He S, Varghese RS, et al. Identification of race-associated metabolite biomarkers for hepatocellular carcinoma in patients with liver cirrhosis and hepatitis C virus infection. PLoS One. 2018;**13**:e0192748

[178] Banales JM, Inarrairaegui M, Arbelaiz A, et al. Serum metabolites as diagnostic biomarkers for cholangiocarcinoma, hepatocellular carcinoma, and primary sclerosing cholangitis. Hepatology. 2018. Available from: https://doi.org/10.1002/hep.30319

[179] Khattab M, Fouad M, Ahmed E. Role of biomarkers in the prediction and diagnosis of hepatocellular carcinoma. World Journal of Hepatology. 2015;**7**:2474-2481

[180] Ferrarini A, Di Poto C, He S, et al. Metabolomic analysis of liver tissues for characterization of hepatocellular carcinoma. Journal of Proteome Research. 2019. DOI: 10.1021/acs.jproteome.9b00185

[181] Ferrin G, Aguilar-Melero P, Rodriguez-Peralvarez M, Montero-Alvarez JL, de la Mata M. Biomarkers for hepatocellular carcinoma: Diagnostic and therapeutic utility. Hepatic Medicine: Evidence And Research. 2015;**7**:1-10

[182] Kelly TK, De Carvalho DD, Jones PA. Epigenetic modifications as therapeutic targets. Nature Biotechnology. 2010;**28**:1069-1078

[183] Vernon G, Baranova A, Younossi ZM. Systematic review: The epidemiology and natural history of non-alcoholic fatty liver disease and non-alcoholic steatohepatitis in adults. Alimentary Pharmacology & Therapeutics. 2011;**34**:274-285

[184] Sumner AE, Cowie CC. Ethnic differences in the ability of triglyceride levels to identify insulin resistance. Atherosclerosis. 2008;**196**:696-703

[185] Sumner AE, Vega GL, Genovese DJ, Finley KB, Bergman RN, Boston RC. Normal triglyceride levels despite insulin resistance in African Americans: Role of lipoprotein lipase. Metabolism. 2005;**54**:902-909

[186] Giannini E, Testa R. The metabolic syndrome: All criteria are equal, but some criteria are more equal than others. Archives of Internal Medicine. 2003;**163**:2787-2788. Author reply 2788

[187] Grohmann M, Wiede F, Dodd GT, et al. Obesity drives STAT-1-dependent NASH and STAT-3-dependent HCC. Cell. 2018;**175**:1289-1306.e20

[188] Nakagawa H, Hayata Y, Kawamura S, Yamada T, Fujiwara N, Koike K. Lipid metabolic reprogramming in hepatocellular carcinoma. Cancers. 2018;**10**:447. DOI: 10.3390/cancers10110447

[189] Noureddin M, Vipani A, Bresee C, et al. NASH leading cause of liver transplant in women: Updated analysis of indications for liver transplant and ethnic and gender variances. The American Journal of Gastroenterology. 2018;**113**:1649-1659

[190] Ruhl CE, Everhart JE. Determinants of the association of overweight with elevated serum alanine aminotransferase activity in the United States. Gastroenterology. 2003;**124**:71-79

[191] Fleischman MW, Budoff M, Zeb I, Li D, Foster T. NAFLD prevalence differs among hispanic subgroups: The multi-ethnic study of atherosclerosis. World Journal of Gastroenterology. 2014;**20**:4987-4993

[192] Neuschwander-Tetri BA, Clark JM, Bass NM, et al. Clinical, laboratory and histological associations in adults with nonalcoholic fatty liver disease. Hepatology. 2010;**52**:913-924

[193] Hosaka T, Suzuki F, Kobayashi M, et al. Long-term entecavir treatment reduces hepatocellular carcinoma incidence in patients with hepatitis B virus infection. Hepatology. 2013;**58**:98-107

[194] Moon AM, Green PK, Berry K, Ioannou GN. Transformation of hepatitis C antiviral treatment in a national healthcare system following the introduction of direct antiviral agents. Alimentary Pharmacology & Therapeutics. 2017;**45**:1201-1212

[195] Tampaki M, Savvanis S, Koskinas J. Impact of direct-acting antiviral agents on the development of hepatocellular carcinoma: Evidence and pathophysiological issues. Annals of Gastroenterology. 2018;**31**:670-679

[196] Barchetta I, Carotti S, Labbadia G, et al. Liver vitamin D receptor, CYP2R1, and CYP27A1 expression: Relationship with liver histology and vitamin D3 levels in patients with nonalcoholic steatohepatitis or hepatitis C virus. Hepatology. 2012;**56**:2180-2187

[197] Eliades M, Spyrou E. Vitamin D: A new player in non-alcoholic fatty liver disease? World Journal of Gastroenterology. 2015;**21**:1718-1727

[198] Beilfuss A, Sowa JP, Sydor S, et al. Vitamin D counteracts fibrogenic

TGF-beta signalling in human hepatic stellate cells both receptor-dependently and independently. Gut. 2015;**64**:791-799

[199] Erhardt A, Stahl W, Sies H, Lirussi F, Donner A, Haussinger D. Plasma levels of vitamin E and carotenoids are decreased in patients with nonalcoholic steatohepatitis (NASH). European Journal of Medical Research. 2011;**16**:76-78

[200] Montella M, Crispo A, Giudice A. HCC, diet and metabolic factors: Diet and HCC. Hepatitis Monthly. 2011;**11**:159-162

[201] Bhat M, Sonenberg N, Gores GJ. The mTOR pathway in hepatic malignancies. Hepatology. 2013;**58**:810-818

[202] Dongiovanni P, Petta S, Mannisto V, et al. Statin use and non-alcoholic steatohepatitis in at risk individuals. Journal of Hepatology. 2015;**63**:705-712

Section 4

New Diagnostic Tools for Nonalcoholic Fatty Liver Disease

Chapter 6

Current Noninvasive MR-Based Imaging Methods in Assessing NAFLD Patients

Diana Feier, Delia Muntean, Nina Bastati and Ahmed Ba-Ssalamah

Abstract

The chapter will focus on the different aspects of nonalcoholic fatty liver disease (NAFLD). An update in noninvasive MR-based imaging will be offered in detail, pointing mainly to fat, iron, and fibrosis deposition and the accuracy of quantitative methods in disease grading and severity assessment. NAFLD is the most common cause of chronic liver disease (CLD) in Western countries. MRI is used to evaluate the disease, to assess the severity, and to quantify the amount of fat deposition, being also the method of choice to evaluate and quantify iron overload. Diagnosis and staging of liver fibrosis is one of the most challenging aspects of non-invasive imaging. "Virtual biopsy" refers to the possibility of imaging techniques to depict, map, and measure fibrosis minimizing the need for invasive liver biopsies in CLD. MRI allows an accurate determination of steatosis, iron overload, and fibrosis, even if they coexist.

Keywords: steatosis, fibrosis, iron overload, contrast-enhanced MRI, chemical shift sequences

1. Introduction

1.1 The importance of noninvasive evaluation of liver steatosis and fibrosis in NAFLD patients

NAFLD is currently the most common cause of CLD worldwide. It is defined by lipid droplet accumulation within hepatocytes in the absence of substantial alcohol intake. NAFLD comprises a disease spectrum ranging from simple steatosis to nonalcoholic steatohepatitis (NASH), which may progress into liver fibrosis and even end-stage cirrhosis [1]. NAFLD is becoming a major concern with the increasing incidence of obesity in Europe. Available data suggest that the global prevalence of NAFLD is estimated at 24%, being the leading cause of CLD in the USA and Europe [2].

The differentiation of simple steatosis from NASH has a great clinical importance. Additionally to liver steatosis, NASH presents inflammation and hepatocellular injury [3]. The differentiation between both entities is routinely made by histopathological analysis after liver biopsy. However, it is an invasive method, with inherent risks that include sampling error and serious complications [4].

IntechOpen

Currently, there is an urgent need for a noninvasive method to accurately assess liver fibrosis and liver steatosis. Ultrasonography (US)-based and computer tomography (CT)-based modalities can demonstrate the morphologic alterations of cirrhosis, but they are limited in evaluating patients with earlier stages of liver disease [5].

Advancements in magnetic resonance imaging (MRI), with its unique and intrinsic imaging features, have provided the opportunity to revolutionize how we image and evaluate patients with diffuse liver diseases. In addition, with the development of new antifibrotic therapeutic agents, MRI-based techniques may play a central role in monitoring treatment response and in the clinical management of patients with NAFLD [6, 7].

The recent technical developments in MRI hardware and software, including the use of three Tesla MR devices in daily routine work, have significantly improved the temporal and spatial resolutions, especially in the case of contrast-enhanced T1-weighted 3D sequences. The use of various liver-specific hepatobiliary contrast agents enables not only morphological characterization but also a functional assessment of all liver lesions and also characterization of diffuse parenchymal changes [8].

2. Liver biopsy: the available but imperfect gold standard

Currently, liver biopsy is the reference standard for the diagnosis and staging of liver fibrosis [4]. However, this procedure has several major limitations, including its invasive nature, risk for potential complications, poor patient acceptance, interobserver variability, and possible sampling errors [4, 9].

Liver biopsy captures only a tiny fraction of the liver (roughly 1/50.000), leading to sampling errors [10]. In an attempt to reduce sampling variability, it is recommended that liver biopsy specimens be at least 2.0 cm long and contain at least 11 portal triads. Biopsy specimens that do not meet these criteria are associated with a high risk of under staging (false negative) [11].

In contrast to fibrosis in chronic viral hepatitis, fibrosis in alcoholic hepatitis and in the adult form of NAFLD begins adjacent to the central veins. The fibrosis is laid down in a perisinusoidal manner, and the scar tissue surrounds individual hepatocytes. As the disease advances, perisinusoidal fibrosis accumulates adjacent to portal tracts, and the fibrotic tissue eventually coalesces into fibrous bridges connecting portal triads and central veins, ultimately culminating in cirrhosis [3]. As cirrhosis develops, the characteristic histologic features of fatty liver disease may be lost. The perisinusoidal may no longer be apparent, and other features (e.g., inflammatory cells, ballooned hepatocytes, and steatosis) may subside. Thus, cirrhosis due to fatty liver disease may be indistinguishable from cirrhosis due to viral hepatitis or other causes [12].

3. MRI-based methods for the noninvasive diagnosis of NAFLD

The search for the best diagnostic technique in terms of noninvasiveness and accuracy is still a major concern in recent research activity. In the recent literature, the role of several imaging diagnosis tools and specific contrast agents is reported in the evaluation of diffuse liver diseases such as steatosis, fibrosis, and cirrhosis.

The differentiation of prognostically relatively benign simple steatosis from potentially progressive NASH is a crucial issue [13, 14]. Moreover, NAFLD is a reversible condition, especially during the early onset of the disease; therefore diagnosing and correct staging of patients with NAFLD are essential in order to prevent the development of an irreversible advanced liver disease.

Routine biochemical laboratory tests and conventional imaging, including US, CT, and non-specific gadolinium-enhanced MRI, cannot distinguish between these entities with sufficient confidence [15, 16]. Therefore, the differentiation between both entities is routinely made by histopathological analysis after liver biopsy. Liver biopsy is still considered the reference standard for the diagnosis of NASH [4]. There are several histological scoring systems to grade NASH, and the most commonly used is the so-called NAFLD activity score (NAS) [17]. The steatosis activity and fibrosis score (SAF) are a newly developed system for categorizing liver histology in NAFLD patients [18]. The lack of reliable, noninvasive methods for the diagnosis of disease severity and prediction of prognosis is one of the major drawbacks in the clinical management of patients with NAFLD [19].

3.1 The diagnostic value of MR imaging techniques in assessing NAFLD

3.1.1 Magnetic resonance elastography

Magnetic resonance elastography (MRE) assesses viscoelastic properties of soft tissues [20], offering a direct insight into the liver parenchymal stiffness. First step in the MRE technique is generating mechanical waves in the liver tissue. Then gradient-echo sequences are used to image wave motion, while a specialized software utilizing inversion algorithms transforms the images obtained into elastograms, revealing the tissues' stiffness quantitative map, expressed in kilopascals [21].

Studies comparing healthy volunteers and patients with CLD established that the shear viscoelastic parameters of the liver increased according to the stage of liver fibrosis, and a statistically significant difference between the patients with Metavir scores F0–F1 fibrosis versus F2–F3, F2–F3 versus F4, and F0–F1 versus F4 was found [20, 22]. MRE also proved to be superior to biochemical testing using the aspartate aminotransferase-to-platelet ratio index [22]. Most importantly the authors could clearly separate the intermediate fibrosis stages, using MRE elasticity measurements.

Chen et al. [23] demonstrated that MRE-based assessments of liver stiffness in patients with NAFLD may have a high diagnostic accuracy (AUC 0.93) for discriminating NASH from simple steatosis, with a cutoff value of 2.74 kPa reaching 94% sensitivity and 73% specificity. However, a more recent study suggested that the performance of MRE for diagnosis of NASH versus simple steatosis was rather modest and did not provide a high level of accuracy. Using 2D-MRE (60 Hz), 3D-MRE (60 Hz), and 3D-MRE (40 Hz), the AUROC for diagnosing definite NASH was 0.754, 0.757, and 0.736, respectively [24].

In a prospective study, Cui et al. [25] proved that the diagnostic accuracy of 2D-MRE for the noninvasive evaluation of advanced fibrosis in patients with biopsy-proven NAFLD was significantly higher than five clinical prediction rules, widely validated for the assessment of fibrosis in patients with NAFLD, such as the NAFLD fibrosis score, the BARD score, the AST-to-ALT ratio, FIB-4, and AST-to-platelet ratio index. Using the cutoff value for 2D-MRE of 3.64 kPa, the AUROC of 2D-MRE for predicting advanced fibrosis was 0.957. This proved to be significantly higher than FIB-4 score with AUROC of 0.861, the best-of-all analyzed clinical prediction rules. Therefore, 2D-MRE is a promising noninvasive imaging-based biomarker for the diagnosis of advanced fibrosis in NAFLD patients used additionally to clinical prediction rules, especially when the latter have indeterminate values.

The cutoff values proposed by Loomba et al. [26] for the prediction of each fibrosis stage using 2D-SWE in patients with NAFLD were 3.02 kPa for early fibrosis, 3.58 kPa for significant fibrosis, 3.64 kPa for advanced fibrosis, and 4.67 kPa for the prediction of cirrhosis, with areas under the ROC curve of 0.838,

0.856, 0.924, and 0.894, respectively. The most promising results were obtained for discriminating advanced fibrosis (F3–F4) from fibrosis stages 0–2 with a sensitivity of 0.86 (95% confidence interval [CI]: 0.65–0.97) and a specificity of 0.91 (95% CI, 0.83–0.96).

Kim et al. showed, however, that the best cutoff for detecting advanced fibrosis value was 4.15 kPa (AUROC = 0.954, sensitivity = 85%, specificity = 92%). The performance of this technique for discriminating between other fibrosis stages was also satisfactory [27].

Nevertheless, this ability to stage pre-cirrhotic disease could make MRE very useful for the assessment of therapeutic success and disease progression [28].

More advanced versions of the imaging modality such as 3D-MRE allow the evaluation of a larger volume of liver parenchyma than 2D-MRE, being significantly more accurate for diagnosis of advanced fibrosis in NAFLD patients [24].

As it is not affected by the absence of an ultrasound window, MRE is more precise than ultrasonographic elastographic techniques. In patients with obesity to morbid obesity, MRE proved to have a better success rate than vibrant-controlled transient elastography (95.8 versus 81.3%) and a higher interobserver agreement than liver biopsy (intraclass correlation coefficient, 0.95 versus 0.89) [29].

Acute inflammation, passive liver congestion caused by cardiac insufficiency, or obstructive cholestasis leads to a false increase of liver stiffness values [30]. Moreover, on a gradient-echo MRE sequence, certain conditions such as iron overload states may lead to a lower MRI signal intensity, which does not allow shear wave recognition. This leads to a decrease in MRE diagnostic accuracy. Thus, using spin-echo or echo-planar sequences with lower T2* effect susceptibility can alleviate this problem [30].

The technique has the advantage of not being influenced by the patient's weight or the presence of ascites. MRE remains expensive and not widely accessible in the everyday imaging routine of patients with NAFLD.

3.1.2 Magnetic resonance spectroscopy

MR spectroscopy (MRS) enables the noninvasive measurement of concentrations of different chemical components within tissues, which are displayed as a 1D spectrum with peaks consistent with the various chemicals detected. The major problem in obtaining MRS signals from abdominal organs is sensitivity to physiologic movement during the scan time usually exceeding several minutes [31]. Usually, the measurement is performed by manually placing a single voxel into the liver parenchyma far from the liver capsule, in an area free of large vessels or bile ducts [32].

While proton MRS is a very useful technique for the quantification of hepatic fat, its use for the estimation of hepatic fibrosis appears to be limited [33, 34].

According to Abrigo et al. [34], phosphorus-MRS (31P-MRS) shows distinct biochemical changes in different NAFLD states and has fair diagnostic accuracy for NASH. However, this technique requires considerable operator skills (sequence programming, shimming, analysis of spectra) and access to special equipment (scanner, 31P coil) [28].

31P-MRS permits in vivo evaluation of energy metabolism and intracellular compartment division through different signals and provides metabolic information, which is useful when assessing fibrogenesis [28]. A significant correlation between phosphodiester concentration and the stage of fibrosis and a correlation between "anabolic charge" (phosphomonoester/[phosphomonoester + phosphodiester]) and the stage of fibrosis were found in a study comparing a group of patients with steatosis and no to moderate inflammation to a group of patients with severe fibrosis or cirrhosis [35].

Hydrogen 1 MRS (1H-MRS) has proven its efficiency in quantifying liver steatosis, by measuring lipid peaks, identified in the liver at 0.9, 1.3, 2.0, 2.2, and 5.3 parts per million. The dominant lipid peaks are caused by the resonance of methyl (-CH3) protons and methylene (-CH2) in the triglyceride molecule [36].

The absolute fat concentration can be therefore calculated using the following formula:

$$\text{Triglyceride content} = \text{total lipid peak area}/(\text{total lipid resonance peak} + \text{water resonance peak}) \quad (1)$$

As the steatosis grade increases, the size of the lipid peaks relative to the water peak increases as well [36].

The advantages of ^{1}H-MRS are the very high sensitivity, a good correlation with histological analysis, and the method's independency of confounders such as fibrosis and iron or glycogen depositions. On the other side, MRS has currently a limited clinical availability, and it is prone to sampling error, when a single-voxel liver spectroscopy is performed [36].

Furthermore, authors assessed the diagnostic accuracy of a novel magnetic resonance protocol for liver tissue characterization, using T1 mapping, 1H spectroscopy, and T2* mapping, which quantified liver fibrosis, steatosis, and hemosiderosis, respectively [37]. According to their results, the novel scanning method provides high diagnostic accuracy for the assessment of all three histology variables.

In a recent study, Idilman et al. [38] analyzed the efficiency of MRI-proton density fat fraction (MRI-PDFF) and MRS-determined liver fat content in patients with NAFLD in comparison with liver biopsy-determined steatosis.

No superiority between the two imaging methods was observed. This study emphasized that the estimation of fat liver content using both MR imaging techniques was more accurate in the absence of liver fibrosis. MRS showed promising results for discriminating moderate/severe steatosis from none/mild steatosis with an AUROC of 0.857. A cutoff value of 9% provided a sensitivity of 92%, negative predictive value of 83.3%, specificity of 71%, and positive predictive value of 84.6%.

The accurate assessment of liver fat content in patients with NAFLD is essential in identifying those who are at greater risk of progressing into advanced fibrosis stages, being also of great value in evaluating the response to therapy. Liver steatosis also influences the successful rate of liver transplantation (LT); one of the necessary requirements in many centers is that the living donor liver must not exceed 5% steatosis, as greater values are associated with increased recipient liver dysfunction [38].

MRS proves to be a highly accurate noninvasive technique, which allows us to distinguish between individuals with simple steatosis and steatohepatitis who may benefit from early intervention and more aggressive therapy.

3.1.3 Diffusion-weighted MR imaging

Diffusion-weighted imaging (DWI) is a noninvasive method that allows measurement of the microscopic motion of water in tissue and generates representative apparent diffusion coefficient (ADC) values. DWI uses very fast scans with an additional series of (diffusion) gradients rapidly turned on and off [28].

Within tissues with highly cellular component and therefore a narrowed extracellular space, the water molecule motion is impeded leading to restricted water diffusion in such tissues. In contrast, fluid-rich or necrotic structures are associated with a greater freedom of motion of water molecules, and the water diffusion in such tissues is considered to be "free." Therefore, on DWI sequences, the signal intensity reflects the tissue diffusion characteristics, which is influenced by cellularity and the integrity of cell membranes [39].

In a prospective study, Guiu et al. [40] demonstrated that both pure molecular diffusion and perfusion-related diffusion were significantly lower in the steatotic liver than in the normal liver. On a group of 89 NAFLD patients who underwent liver biopsy, Murphy et al. [41] also found a good correlation between histologic features of NAFLD liver and DWI-derived quantitative measures. Molecular diffusivity was significantly decreased with steatosis, while perfusion fraction decreased with fibrosis degree. Same associations were found between pediatric NAFLD histologic features and DWI parameters, with a high interobserver reproducibility [42]. As far as the apparent diffusion coefficient is concerned, studies show inconsistent results. One study in adults with NAFLD found that ADC decreased with steatosis, while others found no significant relationship [40, 41].

Several studies have evaluated the use of DWI and ADC values for the diagnosis of hepatic fibrosis or cirrhosis in patients with diffuse hepatopathies. The complex assembly of collagen fibers, glycosaminoglycan, and proteoglycans that constitutes liver fibrosis may restrict the molecular diffusion measured by DWI [43].

DWI has been successfully applied to differentiate cirrhotic from healthy tissue. Girometti et al. reported a positive predictive value of 100%, a negative predictive value of 99.9%, and an overall accuracy of 96.4% in cirrhotic patients compared to healthy controls [44].

A recent meta-analysis suggests that DWI parameters can reliably stage hepatic fibrosis, having a good diagnostic accuracy with areas under the SROC curve between 80 and 90%. A high *b* value for liver fibrosis imaging (between 800 and 1000 s/mm^2) could significantly increase the diagnostic accuracy of diffusion imaging in differentiating between significant and severe fibroses (>F2). For diagnosing liver cirrhosis (F4), the use of 3T MRI equipment has also proved to optimize the DWI diagnostic accuracy, compared to 2T MRI [45].

Lewin et al. found a significant relationship between the ADC values and necroinflammatory scores and suspected an influence of steatosis on apparent diffusion coefficient values [46]. In addition, the ADC of fibrotic livers was decreased as the fibrosis scores increased in some studies [46], but not in others [43].

However, differences in MR equipment and sequence parameters make it difficult to compare studies. Clearly, more research is needed to create a standard setup for DWI sequence acquisition to make studies comparable and to determine whether or not DWI can be a useful tool for the diagnosis and staging of diffuse liver diseases.

Furthermore, DWI imaging is susceptible to artifacts (e.g., blurring, ghosting, and distortions) and offers a limited image quality; therefore, DWI is currently used as complementary and not as a replacement to conventional sequences in the evaluation of NAFLD [47].

DWI does not require administration of intravenous contrast; consequently the technique might represent a reasonable option for patients with kidney failure, where gadolinium-based contrast substances represent a contraindication due to the increased risk of developing nephrogenic systemic fibrosis, while iodinated CT contrast might lead to an even greater impairment of renal function, being also contraindicated [47].

3.1.4 Susceptibility-weighted MR imaging

It is known that, among other factors, increased iron content of the liver and secondary changes manifesting in progressive collagen deposition are important background alterations in the development of liver fibrosis [48].

Susceptibility-weighted imaging (SWI) is well known as a three-dimensional (3D) gradient-echo (GRE) technique utilizing phase information to increase sensitivity for detecting susceptibility changes that result from, for example, iron, hemoglobin, and calcification. Initially used for neuroimaging [49, 50], recent technical advances allow for possible abdominal applications.

SWI is based on T2*-weighted GRE sequences and exploits both magnitude and phase information. Traditionally SWI sequences are high-resolution 3D sequences. Employing 3D sequences for abdominal imaging is not feasible because of long acquisition times and the large B0 variations encountered in this body area. With the advent of a multi-breath-hold GRE-sequence-based SWI, a two-dimensional (2D) sequence was developed for abdominal imaging [51]. SWI utilizes the differences in the magnetic susceptibilities of different tissues and produces a contrast superior to conventional T1- and T2-weighted MR imaging in the detection of structures that cause susceptibility artifacts [52].

The superiority of SWI over the T2*-weighted sequence has been shown, both in the detection and conspicuity of increased liver iron deposition and siderotic nodules [51] and in the detection of intratumoral hemorrhage in hepatocellular carcinoma (HCC) [53].

The liver-to-muscle signal intensity ratio on SWI proved to be a reliable measurement in grading liver fibrosis in patient with diffuse liver disease, with a high-diagnostic accuracy for the differentiation of moderate to advanced (F2 and F3) liver fibrosis from liver cirrhosis (F4) (AUROC = 0.93). The multiple regression analysis showed that liver fibrosis independently influenced SWI measurements, being a main contributor to the decreasing liver-to-muscle SI ratio, followed by iron overload and necroinflammatory activity, when compared with histopathologic findings [52].

The relationship between iron load and fibrogenesis has multiple considerations. The increased iron content in the liver, either diffusely distributed or in the form of numerous siderotic nodules, does not represent the entire transformation of liver fibrosis. In the process of fibrogenesis, hepatic stellate cells are also activated by other factors such as inflammation, genetic determinants, and the immune system [52].

Using a multiparametric approach, a recent study proved that liver SWI signal intensity enhanced the diagnostic performance in diagnosing and staging liver fibrosis, when used together with the apparent diffusion coefficient of the liver parenchyma on DWI and the degree of liver enhancement on the hepatobiliary phase of dynamic contrast-enhanced MRI. The three MRI techniques used together were able to assess the severity of liver fibrosis with an AUC ranging from 0.90 to 0.95, and the best performance was obtained in predicting moderate fibrosis (F2 or greater), with a sensitivity of 86% and a specificity of 94%. This reflects the clinical significance of this diagnostic tool, as F2 or greater is the stage in which therapeutic action should be taken [54].

3.1.5 Proton density fat fraction

Proton density fat fraction (PDFF) measurement is a multi-echo chemical shift-encoded MRI method for quantitatively assessing hepatic steatosis, being available as an option from several manufacturers of MRI scanners. PDFF is defined as the ratio of the density of mobile protons from triglycerides and the total density of protons from mobile triglycerides and mobile water. It is expressed as an absolute percentage (%) and ranges from 0 to 100% [7].

This sequence allows the measurement of fat fraction in any segment of the liver, generating a fat mapping of the entire hepatic parenchyma. This is of great value, as several studies proved the heterogeneous intrahepatic fat distribution [55].

The advantages of PDFF calculation are its ability to be completely obtained during a short breath-hold (in less than 25 s) and the fact that it minimizes the errors from confounders of fat quantification encountered using conventional MRI methods (Dixon and fat saturation) such as T1 bias, T2* decay, or spectral complexity of lipid [38].

Emerging data support the use of MRI-PDFF in evaluating the response to treatment in the setting of early-phase clinical trials in NASH, using drugs with an anti-steatotic mechanism of action [7].

In a recent study, the mean fat fraction was significantly lower in the left lobe than it was in the right, while liver segments 4 and 5 proved to be the most adequate to estimate the entire hepatic lipid content [55].

Regarding technical parameters, using a six-echo map proved to have a higher diagnostic accuracy than three, four, or five echoes [56].

Permutt et al. showed a good correlation between MRI-PDFF and histology-determined steatosis grade in adults with NAFLD. They observed an increasing average value of MRI-determined PDFF with increasing steatosis grade (8.9% for grade 1, 16.3% for grade 2, and 25% for grade 3 steatoses) [57]. PDFF was effective in differentiating moderate or severe hepatic steatosis from mild or no hepatic steatosis, with area under the curve of 0.95 and 93% sensitivity and 85% specificity. However, the correlation between biopsy and PDFF-determined steatosis was less pronounced when fibrosis was present ($r = 0.60$) than when fibrosis was absent [58].

When comparing the efficiency of MRI-PDFF to magnetic resonance spectroscopy, both techniques proved to strongly correlate with the histology-determined steatosis, with no superiority between them [38]. But the PDFF maps have the advantage of being automatically reconstructed without user input or post-processing, unlike MR spectroscopy-based methods.

Therefore, MR-PDFF represents another novel, noninvasive, and practical imaging tool in assessing patients with NAFLD, as the entire liver can be covered in assessment with a great accuracy in quantifying total hepatic fat amount [38, 55].

3.1.6 Contrast-enhanced MRI

In the liver, contrast agents are categorized into non-specific agents that distribute into the vascular and extravascular extracellular spaces (such as the linear gadopentetate dimeglumine (Gd-DTPA) and the macrocyclic gadobutrol (Gd-DO3A-butrol) and gadoterate dimeglumine (Gd-DOTA)) and liver-specific agents taken up by liver cells. These liver-specific agents are either taken up by Kupffer cells (such as the super paramagnetic iron oxide particles ferumoxides and ferucarbotran) or by hepatocytes (such as gadolinium ethoxybenzyl dimeglumine or gadoxetic acid (Gd-EOB-DTPA) and gadobenate dimeglumine (Gd-BOPTA)) [8].

3.1.6.1 Hepato-specific contrast-enhanced MRI

Gadoxetic acid (Gd-EOB-DTPA, Eovist® in the USA, Primovist® in Europe) is a liver-specific MRI contrast agent which provides both morphological and functional information and can be used as an imaging biomarker in the diagnostic workup of liver fibrosis [8].

After intravenous injection, the gadoxetic acid (GA) distributes into the vascular and extravascular spaces during the arterial, portal venous, and late dynamic phases and progressively into the hepatocytes and bile ducts during the hepatobiliary phase. GA enhancement depends mainly on liver perfusion, vascular permeability, extracellular diffusion, and hepatocyte transporter expression [8, 59].

All these functions are disturbed in diffuse liver diseases, and there may be a decrease in the balance between uptake and excretion of the contrast media by the impaired hepatocytes.

The transport of GA in the hepatocytes is mediated by two different transport systems located at the sinusoidal and canalicular membranes of the cell [60]. The contrast agent enters the hepatocytes through two organic anion-transporting polypeptide transporters (OATP1B1 and OATP1B3) [61], and it is excreted into the bile via the multidrug resistance protein 2 (MRP2) [62].

In patients with liver cirrhosis, the upregulation of MRP2 is associated with significant signal loss on gadoxetic acid-enhanced MR images [63]. Organic acid efflux from hepatocytes may also occur through the sinusoidal membrane because the transport through OATP is bidirectional and because the sinusoidal membrane also contains multidrug resistance proteins (MRP3 and MRP4), as it is illustrated in **Figure 1**. These efflux pumps are normally expressed at low levels in normal hepatocytes but can be upregulated in pathologic conditions, such as cholestasis. GA is not metabolized within hepatocytes [64].

With GA, approximately 50% of the administered dose in the normal human liver is transported through the hepatocytes and excreted into the bile, and the percentage of the contrast agent that is not cleared by the hepatobiliary system is excreted by glomerular filtration in the kidneys [65].

Hepatobiliary MR contrast agents can be used to characterize liver functional properties, and the relative enhancement quantification is a reflection of hepatocyte malfunction as a result of liver fibrosis accumulation and increased necroinflammatory activity [66].

Several MR-derived parameters can be used to estimate the amount of GA uptake, such as the relative liver enhancement, hepatic uptake index, and T1 mapping during hepatobiliary phase—on static images or the hepatic extraction fraction and liver blood flow—by using dynamic assessment [67]. Importantly, there is currently no clear consensus as to which of these MR-derived parameters is the most suitable for assessing liver dysfunction.

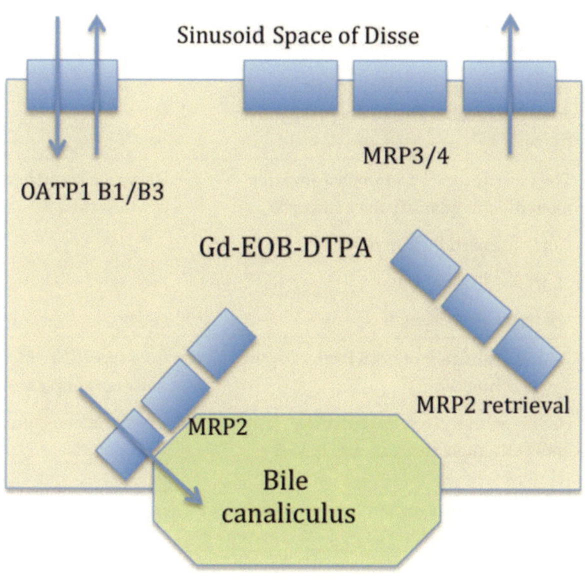

Figure 1.
Cellular pharmacology of Gd-EOB-DTPA—figure adapted after Van Beers et al. [8].

The relative liver enhancement (RLE), the most commonly used parameter, is calculated by subtracting the signal intensity (SI) on the unenhanced images from the SI in the HBP, and dividing the difference by the SI of the unenhanced images, using the following formula [67]:

$$\text{Relative enhancement (RE)} = (\text{SI 20 minutes post - contrast - SI pre - contrast})/\text{SI pre - contrast} \quad (2)$$

In order to avoid bias due to liver parenchyma inhomogeneity, several regions of interest (ROI) are placed in different segments of both liver lobes.

Indeed, reports on animal models also proved that gadoxetic acid-enhanced MRI could differentiate simple steatosis from NASH by comparing the signal profile or the time of maximum relative enhancement [68]. Furthermore, several recent

Imaging technique	Advantages	Disadvantages
MRE	• Excellent diagnostic accuracy for staging liver fibrosis and cirrhosis • Uninfluenced by obesity or ascites	• Increased failure rate in iron overload states • Not widely available
MRS	• Excellent sensitivity for detecting mild steatosis • Good correlation with histological analysis • Independent of confounders (e.g., fibrosis, iron, glycogen)	• Requires specialized post-processing data, expensive • Sensitive to field inhomogeneity • Technical limitations: low signal-to-noise ratio, motion • Evaluation of small portion of the liver
DWI	• Functional information in the absence of intravenous contrast • Successfully applied to differentiate cirrhotic from healthy tissue	• Limited image quality • Susceptible to artifacts (e.g., blurring, ghosting, and distortions) • Needs further research
SWI	• Iron overload quantification • Enhances the diagnostic performance of other MRI techniques in diagnosing liver fibrosis	• Susceptibility artifacts
PDFF	• The most accurate and precise imaging biomarker to quantify liver steatosis • Not influenced by iron overload • Short acquisition time • Volumetric assessment	• Accuracy could be affected by fibrosis, severe steatosis
Liver-specific contrast MRI	• Allows evaluation of both liver morphology and function • High sensitivity in differentiating between simple steatosis and NASH	• Low specificity in differentiating between simple steatosis and NASH • Confounders: increased liver function parameters

MRE, magnetic resonance elastography; MRS, magnetic resonance spectroscopy; DWI, diffusion-weighted MR imaging; SWI, susceptibility-weighted MR imaging; PDFF, proton density fat fraction.

Table 1.
Summary of main advantages and disadvantages of different MRI techniques in evaluating patients with NAFLD.

studies have shown the ability of gadoxetic acid-enhanced MRI to evaluate patients with CLD, particularly for the staging of hepatic fibrosis, and to obtain global and territorial liver function information [69].

In a retrospective, proof-of-concept study, the mean relative enhancement of the whole liver after GA administration was significantly lower in patients with NASH (0.82 ± 0.22), compared to those with simple steatosis (1.39 ± 0.52) [70]. Therefore, the relative enhancement measurements could potentially be used to differentiate between simple steatosis and NASH [AUC = 0.85 (95% CI 0.75–0.91)], providing a high sensitivity of 97% but a low specificity of 63% [70].

Histology parameters used to stage NASH, such as lobular inflammation, hepatocellular ballooning, and the degree of liver fibrosis, proved to be independent factors that negatively correlated with RLE. On the other side, fatty liver infiltration did not correlate with the relative enhancement. Due to its low specificity, GA-MRI cannot be used at this moment as the only criterion by which to differentiate simple steatosis and NASH. However, GA-MRI can be used as a valuable screening tool in identifying which NAFLD patients need to perform liver biopsy and which do not [70].

With regard to liver fibrosis staging, the contrast enhancement index (method that uses the paraspinal muscles' signal intensity as a reference for liver) proved to be an efficient biomarker, with higher diagnostic accuracy than other enhancement parameters or hematologic markers [71]. RLE is best suited for detecting moderate to advanced fibrosis, but the interpretation of results should consider laboratory parameters, with special attention to liver function. Elevated levels of aspartate aminotransferase, gammaglutamyl transpeptidase, and alkaline phosphatase levels were independent predictors of false-negative results [69].

The main advantages and disadvantages of each magnetic resonance imaging technique currently used in the noninvasive assessment of NAFLD are briefly synthetized in **Table 1**.

4. Conclusion

MRI is currently increasingly used in the assessment of NAFLD. Although all methods have their own advantages and disadvantages, the noninvasive diagnosis of NAFLD using innovative applications of MRI-based methods presents a promising future. Liver fibrosis can be accurately assessed using MRI methods that do not require contrast media administration, such as MRE, diffusion-weighted MRI, and susceptibility-weighted MRI, while quantitative detection of liver steatosis is better performed using MRS or chemical shift-based MRI techniques such as proton density fat fraction. Moreover, GA-enhanced MRI provides both morphological and functional information and can be used as an imaging biomarker in the diagnostic workup of liver fibrosis and may help to distinguish between the two subgroups of NAFLD, simple steatosis and nonalcoholic steatohepatitis.

List of abbreviations

ADC	Apparent diffusion coefficient
CLD	Chronic liver disease
CT	Computer tomography
DWI	Diffusion-weighted imaging
GA	Gadoxetic acid
GRE	Gradient echo
LT	Liver transplantation

MRE	Magnetic resonance elastography
PDFF	Proton density fat fraction
MRI	Magnetic resonance imaging
MRP2	Multidrug resistance protein 2
MRS	Magnetic resonance spectroscopy
NAFLD	Nonalcoholic fatty liver disease
NASH	Nonalcoholic steatohepatitis
RLE	Relative liver enhancement
ROI	Region of interest
SI	Signal intensity
SWI	Susceptibility-weighted imaging
US	Ultrasonography

Conflict of interest

There is none to declare.

Author details

Diana Feier[1*], Delia Muntean[2], Nina Bastati[3] and Ahmed Ba-Ssalamah[3]

1 Department of Radiology, Medical University of Cluj-Napoca, Cluj-Napoca, Romania

2 Department of Radiology, "Leon Daniello" Pneumology Clinical Hospital, Cluj-Napoca, Romania

3 Department of Biomedical Imaging and Image-guided Therapy, Medical University of Vienna, Austria

*Address all correspondence to: diana.feier@gmail.com

IntechOpen

© 2019 The Author(s). Licensee IntechOpen. This chapter is distributed under the terms of the Creative Commons Attribution License (http://creativecommons.org/licenses/by/3.0), which permits unrestricted use, distribution, and reproduction in any medium, provided the original work is properly cited.

References

[1] Adams LA, Lindor KD. Nonalcoholic fatty liver disease. Annals of Epidemiology. 2007;**17**(11):863-869

[2] Younossi ZM, Koenig AB, Abdelatif D, Fazel Y, Henry L, Wymer M. Global epidemiology of nonalcoholic fatty liver disease-meta-analytic assessment of prevalence, incidence, and outcomes. Hepatology. 2016;**64**(1):73-84

[3] Yeh MM, Brunt EM. Pathology of nonalcoholic fatty liver disease. American Journal of Clinical Pathology. 2007;**128**(5):837-847

[4] Bravo AA, Sheth SG, Chopra S. Liver biopsy. New England Journal of Medicine. 2001;**344**(7):495-500

[5] van Werven JR, Marsman HA, Nederveen AJ, Smits NJ, ten Kate FJ, van Gulik TM, et al. Assessment of hepatic steatosis in patients undergoing liver resection: Comparison of US, CT, T1-weighted dual-echo MR imaging, and point-resolved 1H MR spectroscopy. Radiology. 2010;**256**:159-168

[6] Hardy T, McPherson S. Imaging-based assessment of steatosis, inflammation and fibrosis in NAFLD. Current Hepatology Reports. 2017;**16**:298-307

[7] Caussy C, Reeder SB, Sirlin CB, Loomba R. Non-invasive, quantitative assessment of liver fat by MRI-PDFF as an endpoint in NASH trials. Hepatology. 2018;**68**(2):763-772

[8] Van Beers BE, Pastor CM, Hussain HK. Primovist, eovist: What to expect? Journal of Hepatology. 2012;**57**(2):421-429

[9] Cadranel JF, Rufat P, Degos F. Practices of liver biopsy in France: Results of a prospective nationwide survey. For the Group of Epidemiology of the French Association for the Study of the Liver (AFEF). Hepatology. 2000;**32**(3):477-481

[10] Regev A, Berho M, Jeffers LJ, Milikowski C, Molina EG, Pyrsopoulos NT, et al. Sampling error and intraobserver variation in liver biopsy in patients with chronic HCV infection. The American Journal of Gastroenterology. 2002;**97**(10):2614-2618

[11] Colloredo G, Guido M, Sonzogni A, Leandro G. Impact of liver biopsy size on histological evaluation of chronic viral hepatitis: The smaller the sample, the milder the disease. Journal of Hepatology. 2003;**39**(2):239-244

[12] Faria SC, Ganesan K, Mwangi I, Shiehmorteza M, Viamonte B, Mazhar S, et al. MR imaging of liver fibrosis: Current state of the art. Radiographics. 2009;**29**(6):1615-1635. A review publication of the Radiological Society of North America, Inc

[13] Nascimbeni F, Pais R, Bellentani S, Day CP, Ratziu V, Loria P, et al. From NAFLD in clinical practice to answers from guidelines. Journal of Hepatology. 2013;**59**(4):859-871

[14] Reid AE. Nonalcoholic steatohepatitis. Gastroenterology. 2001;**121**(3):710-723

[15] Lall CG, Aisen AM, Bansal N, Sandrasegaran K. Nonalcoholic fatty liver disease. American Journal of Roentgenology. 2008;**190**(4):993-1002

[16] Afdhal NH, Curry M. Technology evaluation: A critical step in the clinical utilization of novel diagnostic tests for liver fibrosis. Journal of Hepatology. 2007;**46**(4):543-545

[17] Brunt EM, Kleiner DE, Wilson LA, Belt P, Neuschwander-Tetri BA. Nonalcoholic fatty liver disease

(NAFLD) activity score and the histopathologic diagnosis in NAFLD: Distinct clinicopathologic meanings. Hepatology. 2011;**53**(3):810-820

[18] Bedossa P, Poitou C, Veyrie N, Bouillot JL, Basdevant A, Paradis V, et al. Histopathological algorithm and scoring system for evaluation of liver lesions in morbidly obese patients. Hepatology. 2012;**56**(5):1751-1759

[19] Dowman JK, Tomlinson JW, Newsome PN. Systematic review: The diagnosis and staging of non-alcoholic fatty liver disease and non-alcoholic steatohepatitis. Alimentary Pharmacology & Therapeutics. 2011;**33**(5):525-540

[20] Wang Y, Ganger DR, Levitsky J, Sternick LA, McCarthy RJ, Chen ZE, et al. Assessment of chronic hepatitis and fibrosis: Comparison of MR elastography and diffusion-weighted imaging. American Journal of Roentgenology. 2011;**196**(3):553-561

[21] Venkatesh SK, Yin M, Ehman RL. Magnetic resonance elastography of liver: Technique, analysis, and clinical applications. Journal of Magnetic Resonance Imaging. 2013;**37**:544-555

[22] Huwart L, Sempoux C, Salameh N, Jamart J, Annet L, Sinkus R, et al. Liver fibrosis: Noninvasive assessment with MR elastography versus aspartate aminotransferase-to-platelet ratio index. Radiology. 2007;**245**(2):458-466

[23] Chen J, Talwalkar JA, Yin M, Glaser KJ, Sanderson SO, Ehman RL. Early detection of nonalcoholic steatohepatitis in patients with nonalcoholic fatty liver disease by using MR elastography. Radiology. 2011;**259**(3):749-756

[24] Loomba R, Cui J, Wolfson T, Haufe W, Hooker J, Szeverenyi N, et al. Novel 3D magnetic resonance elastography for the noninvasive diagnosis of advanced fibrosis in NAFLD: A prospective study. The American Journal of Gastroenterology. 2016;**111**(7):986-994

[25] Cui J, Ang B, Haufe W, Hernandez C, Verna EC, Sirlin CB, et al. Comparative diagnostic accuracy of magnetic resonance elastography vs. eight clinical prediction rules for non-invasive diagnosis of advanced fibrosis in biopsy-proven nonalcoholic fatty liver disease: A prospective study. Alimentary Pharmacology & Therapeutics. 2015;**41**:1271-1280

[26] Loomba R, Wolfson T, Ang B, Hooker J, Behling C, Peterson M, et al. Magnetic resonance elastography predicts advanced fibrosis in patients with nonalcoholic fatty liver disease: A prospective study. Hepatology. 2014;**60**(6):1920-1928

[27] Kim D, Kim WR, Talwalkar JA, Kim HJ, Ehman RL. Advanced fibrosis in nonalcoholic fatty liver disease: Noninvasive assessment with MR elastography. Radiology. 2013;**268**(2):411-419

[28] Bonekamp S, Kamel I, Solga S, Clark J. Can imaging modalities diagnose and stage hepatic fibrosis and cirrhosis accurately? Journal of Hepatology. 2009;**50**(1):17-35

[29] Chen J, Yin M, Talwalkar JA, Oudry J, Glaser KJ, Smyrk TC, et al. Assessment of diagnostic performance of MR elastography (MRE) and vibration-controlled transient elastography (VCTE) for detecting hepatic fibrosis in patients with severe to morbid obesity. Radiology. 2017;**283**:418-428

[30] Low G, Kruse SA, Lomas DJ. General review of magnetic resonance elastography. World Journal of Radiology. 2016;**8**:59-72

[31] Irwan R, Sijens PE, Potze JH, Oudkerk M. Correlation of proton

MR spectroscopy and diffusion tensor imaging. Magnetic Resonance Imaging. 2005;**23**(8):851-858

[32] Karlas T, Petroff D, Garnov N, Böhm S, Tenckhoff H, Wittekind C, et al. Non-invasive assessment of hepatic steatosis in patients with NAFLD using controlled attenuation parameter and 1H-MR spectroscopy. PLoS One. 2014;**9**(3):e91987

[33] Cho SG, Kim MY, Kim HJ, Kim YS, Choi W, Shin SH, et al. Chronic hepatitis: In vivo proton MR spectroscopic evaluation of the liver and correlation with histopathologic findings. Radiology. 2001;**221**(3):740-746

[34] Abrigo JM, Shen J, Wong VW, Yeung DK, Wong GL, Chim AM, et al. Non-alcoholic fatty liver disease: Spectral patterns observed from an in vivo phosphorus magnetic resonance spectroscopy study. Journal of Hepatology. 2014;**60**(4):809-815

[35] Noren B, Lundberg P, Ressner M, Wirell S, Almer S, Smedby O. Absolute quantification of human liver metabolite concentrations by localized in vivo 31P NMR spectroscopy in diffuse liver disease. European Radiology. 2005;**15**(1):148-157

[36] Qayyum A. MR spectroscopy of the liver: Principles and clinical applications. Radiographics. 2009;**29**(6):1653-1664

[37] Banerjee R, Pavlides M, Tunnicliffe EM, Piechnik SK, Sarania N, Philips R, et al. Multiparametric magnetic resonance for the non-invasive diagnosis of liver disease. Journal of Hepatology. 2014;**60**(1):69-77

[38] Idilman IS, Keskin O, Celik A, Savas B, Elhan AH, Idilman R, et al. A comparison of liver fat content as determined by magnetic resonance imaging-proton density fat fraction and MRS versus liver histology in non-alcoholic fatty liver disease. Acta Radiologica. 2016;**57**:271-278

[39] Taouli B, Koh DM. Diffusion-weighted MR imaging of the liver. Radiology. 2010;**254**:47-66

[40] Guiu B, Petit JM, Capitan V, Aho S, Masson D, Lefevre PH, et al. Intravoxel incoherent motion diffusion-weighted imaging in nonalcoholic fatty liver disease: A 3.0-T MR study. Radiology. 2012;**265**:96-103

[41] Murphy P, Hooker J, Ang B, Wolfson T, Gamst A, Bydder M, et al. Associations between histologic features of nonalcoholic fatty liver disease (NAFLD) and quantitative diffusion-weighted MRI measurements in adults. Journal of Magnetic Resonance Imaging. 2015;**41**:1629-1638

[42] Manning P, Murphy P, Wang K, Hooker J, Wolfson T, Middleton MS, et al. Liver histology and diffusion-weighted MRI in children with nonalcoholic fatty liver disease: A MAGNET study. Journal of Magnetic Resonance Imaging. 2017;**46**(4):1149-1158

[43] Aube C, Racineux PX, Lebigot J, Oberti F, Croquet V, Argaud C, et al. Diagnosis and quantification of hepatic fibrosis with diffusion weighted MR imaging: Preliminary results. Journal de Radiologie. 2004;**85**(3):301-306

[44] Girometti R, Furlan A, Bazzocchi M, Soldano F, Isola M, Toniutto P, et al. Diffusion-weighted MRI in evaluating liver fibrosis: A feasibility study in cirrhotic patients. La Radiologia Medica. 2007;**112**(3):394-408

[45] Jiang H, Chen J, Gao R, Huang Z, Wu M, Song B. Liver fibrosis staging with diffusion-weighted imaging: A systematic review and meta-analysis. Abdominal Radiology. 2017;**42**:490-501

[46] Lewin M, Poujol-Robert A, Boelle PY, Wendum D, Lasnier E, Viallon M, et al. Diffusion-weighted magnetic resonance imaging for the assessment of fibrosis in chronic hepatitis C. Hepatology. 2007;**46**(3):658-665

[47] Shenoy-Bhangle A, Baliyan V, Kordbacheh H, Guimaraes AR, Kambadakone A. Diffusion weighted magnetic resonance imaging of liver: Principles, clinical applications and recent updates. World Journal of Hepatology. 2017;**9**(26):1081-1091

[48] Schmeltzer PA, Talwalkar JA. Noninvasive tools to assess hepatic fibrosis: Ready for prime time? Gastroenterology Clinics of North America. 2011;**40**(3):507-521

[49] Haacke EM, Mittal S, Wu Z, Neelavalli J, Cheng YC. Susceptibility-weighted imaging: Technical aspects and clinical applications, part 1. American Journal of Neuroradiology. 2009;**30**(1):19-30

[50] Mittal S, Wu Z, Neelavalli J, Haacke EM. Susceptibility-weighted imaging: Technical aspects and clinical applications, part 2. American Journal of Neuroradiology. 2009;**30**(2):232-252

[51] Chen W, DelProposto Z, Wu D, Wang J, Jiang Q, Xuan S, et al. Improved siderotic nodule detection in cirrhosis with susceptibility-weighted magnetic resonance imaging: A prospective study. PLoS One. 2012;**7**(5):e36454

[52] Balassy C, Feier D, Peck-Radosavljevic M, Wrba F, Witoszynskyj S, Kiefer B, et al. Susceptibility-weighted MR imaging in the grading of liver fibrosis: A feasibility study. Radiology. 2014;**270**(1):149-158

[53] Li RK, Zeng MS, Rao SX, Qiang JW, Dai YM, Ji Y, et al. Using a 2D multibreath-hold susceptibility-weighted imaging to visualize intratumoral hemorrhage of hepatocellular carcinoma at 3T MRI: Correlation with pathology. Journal of Magnetic Resonance Imaging. 2012;**36**(4):900-906

[54] Feier D, Balassy C, Bastati N, Fragner R, Wrba F, Ba-Ssalamah A. The diagnostic efficacy of quantitative liver MR imaging with diffusion-weighted, SWI, and hepato-specific contrast-enhanced sequences in staging liver fibrosis—A multiparametric approach. European Radiology. 2016;**26**(2):539-546

[55] Lee H, Jun DW, Kang B-K, Nam E, Chang M, Kim M, et al. Estimating of hepatic fat amount using MRI proton density fat fraction in a real practice setting. Medicine. 2017;**96**(33):e7778

[56] Heba ER, Desai A, Zand KA, Hamilton G, Wolfson T, Schlein AN, et al. Accuracy and the effect of possible subject-based confounders of magnitudebased MRI for estimating hepatic proton density fat fraction in adults, using MR spectroscopy as reference. Journal of Magnetic Resonance Imaging. 2016;**43**:398-406

[57] Permutt Z, Le T-A, Peterson MR, Seki E, Brenner DA, Sirlin C, et al. Correlation between liver histology and novel magnetic resonance imaging in adult patients with non-alcoholic fatty liver disease–MRI accurately quantifies hepatic steatosis in NAFLD. Alimentary Pharmacology & Therapeutics. 2012;**36**(1):22-29

[58] Idilman IS, Aniktar H, Idilman R, Kabacam G, Savas B, Elhan A, et al. Hepatic steatosis: Quantification by proton density fat fraction with MR imaging versus liver biopsy. Radiology. 2013;**267**:767-775

[59] Geier A, Dietrich CG, Voigt S, Kim SK, Gerloff T, Kullak-Ublick GA, et al. Effects of proinflammatory cytokines on rat organic anion transporters

during toxic liver injury and cholestasis. Hepatology. 2003;**38**(2):345-354

[60] Weinmann HJ, Bauer H, Frenzel T, Muhler A, Ebert W. Mechanism of hepatic uptake of gadoxetate disodium. Academic Radiology. 1996;**3**(Suppl 2): S232-S234

[61] Leonhardt M, Keiser M, Oswald S, Kuhn J, Jia J, Grube M, et al. Hepatic uptake of the magnetic resonance imaging contrast agent Gd-EOB-DTPA: Role of human organic anion transporters. Drug Metabolism and Disposition. 2010;**38**(7):1024-1028

[62] International Transporter C, Giacomini KM, Huang SM, Tweedie DJ, Benet LZ, Brouwer KL, et al. Membrane transporters in drug development. Nature Reviews. Drug Discovery. 2010;**9**(3):215-236

[63] Motosugi U, Ichikawa T, Muhi A, Sano K, Morisaka H, Ichikawa S, et al. Magnetic resonance elastography as a predictor of insufficient liver enhancement on gadoxetic acid-enhanced hepatocyte-phase magnetic resonance imaging in patients with type C hepatitis and Child-Pugh class A disease. Investigative Radiology. 2012;**47**(10):566-570

[64] Kullak-Ublick GA, Stieger B, Meier PJ. Enterohepatic bile salt transporters in normal physiology and liver disease. Gastroenterology. 2004;**126**(1):322-342

[65] Reimer P, Schneider G, Schima W. Hepatobiliary contrast agents for contrast-enhanced MRI of the liver: Properties, clinical development and applications. European Radiology. 2004;**14**(4):559-578

[66] Tsuda N, Matsui O. Cirrhotic rat liver: Reference to transporter activity and morphologic changes in bile canaliculi–gadoxetic acid-enhanced MR imaging. Radiology. 2010;**256**(3):767-773

[67] Ba-Ssalamah A, Bastati N, Wibmer A, Fragner R, Hodge JC, Trauner M, et al. Hepatic gadoxetic acid uptake as a measure of diffuse liver disease: Where are we? Journal of Magnetic Resonance Imaging. 2017;**45**(3):646-659

[68] Tsuda N, Okada M, Murakami T. New proposal for the staging of nonalcoholic steatohepatitis: Evaluation of liver fibrosis on Gd-EOB-DTPA-enhanced MRI. European Journal of Radiology. 2010;**73**(1):137-142

[69] Feier D, Balassy C, Bastati N, Stift J, Badea R, Ba-Ssalamah A. Liver fibrosis: Histopathologic and biochemical influences on diagnostic efficacy of hepatobiliary contrast-enhanced MR imaging in staging. Radiology. 2013;**269**(2):460-468

[70] Bastati N, Feier D, Wibmer A, Traussnigg S, Balassy C, Tamandl D, et al. Noninvasive differentiation of simple steatosis and steatohepatitis by using gadoxetic acid-enhanced MR imaging in patients with nonalcoholic fatty liver disease: A proof-of-concept study. Radiology. 2014;**271**:739-747

[71] Watanabe H, Kanematsu M, Goshima S, Kondo H, Onozuka M, Moriyama N, et al. Staging hepatic fibrosis: Comparison of gadoxetate disodium-enhanced and diffusionweighted MR imaging—Preliminary observations. Radiology. 2011;**259**:142-150